T0163694

I REFUSED CHEMO

I REFUSED CHEMO

7 Steps to Taking Back Your Power
& Healing Your Cancer

TERI DALE

NEW YORK

LONDON • NASHVILLE • MELBOURNE • VANCOUVER

I REFUSED CHEMO
7 Steps to Taking Back Your Power & Healing Your Cancer

© 2018 Teri Dale

All rights reserved. No portion of this book may be reproduced, stored in a retrieval system, or transmitted in any form or by any means—electronic, mechanical, photocopy, recording, scanning, or other—except for brief quotations in critical reviews or articles, without the prior written permission of the publisher.

Published in New York, New York, by Morgan James Publishing in partnership with Difference Press. Morgan James is a trademark of Morgan James, LLC. www.MorganJamesPublishing.com

The Morgan James Speakers Group can bring authors to your live event. For more information or to book an event visit The Morgan James Speakers Group at www.TheMorganJamesSpeakersGroup.com.

ISBN 9781683508038 paperback
ISBN 9781683508045 eBook
Library of Congress Control Number: 2017915899

Cover Design by:
Rachel Lopez
www.r2cdesign.com

Interior Design by:
Christopher Kirk
www.GFSstudio.com

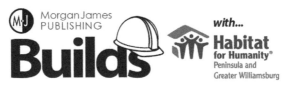

In an effort to support local communities, raise awareness and funds, Morgan James Publishing donates a percentage of all book sales for the life of each book to Habitat for Humanity Peninsula and Greater Williamsburg.

Get involved today! Visit
www.MorganJamesBuilds.com

*For all women struggling with cancer who are
scared and feeling torn:
There is hope. You can get your
power back and heal.*

TABLE OF CONTENTS

FOREWORD

'm not sure if I ever met someone who was both so self-determined and anxious at the same time. Her eyes darted around my office as she wiggled in her chair like someone interviewing for their dream job: excited, yet terrified of rejection. Most of my new patient consults involve me asking most of the questions in an attempt to determine whether I believe I could help them and if they'd be a good fit for the practice. This was different; it was as if I was being interviewed.

To say that Teri Dale is determined is like saying Niagara is just a waterfall. She wanted to find a natural doctor to help her beat her cancer, and losing wasn't an option. Her husband was calm and stalwart, and, though the antithesis of her anxiety, he shared her determined, mind-already-made-up spirit. Again, I felt like the one under the microscope and secretly contemplated that this is the way it always should be.

In the cancer world, patients are often so frightened by their diagnosis. Blindly accepting of their doctor's choice of care, they are herded through the process of surgery, chemotherapy, and radiation before the whirlwind of angst can even settle in their head. It takes the courage of a warrior to cry, "Stop." It was this courage that I found in both Teri and her husband. They were willing to buck the system to search for a better way.

Searching for a better way is what this book is all about. Teri urges her readers to cry, "Stop" just long enough to clear their head and do a little research. Whether one chooses to continue the path with the oncologist or not, adding alternative therapies will increase the chance of the desired outcome.

I wish everyone had the fortitude to push against the pack, but fear is a powerful motivator. Teri's book attempts to remove a little of the panic of cancer. Knowing that others have "beaten it" while keeping their convictions gives strength and hope to everyone with the diagnosis. Perhaps it helps calm the loneliness one experiences. This feeling of isolation in the midst of a crowd may be the most common emotion that cancer patients describe to me. They feel alone. They feel alone in their suffering; alone in their fear; alone in their contemplation of treatment choices.

One of the questions I have on my new patient intake form is, "How supportive is your family?" These few words are powerful, as they reveal the depth of compassion of those you call close. Often, cancer patients are pushed towards standard oncological procedures simply to thrust all responsibility of outcome onto another. "I wish you'd just do what the doctor said to do," is code for, "If I support you in your quest for alternative care, then I take some of the responsibility to help you and I don't want to do that."

People are scared. I understand, but the medical profession is all too happy to take full responsibility for someone's care up until the point of everything going south. They will tell the patient that they are crazy for taking vitamins and that diet has "nothing to do with cancer" while feeding them pudding and donuts during their chemo sessions. Then, if the "cancer returns with a vengeance," they quickly wash their hands of all blame and claim that they did all they could. But did they?

We are all going to die someday, but may it not be of ignorance! Neither may it be of solely trusting in some oncologist that has but three tools in his tool bag. God gave us each a brain and He expects us to use it, as difficult as that may sometimes be. Do your research, read books, watch videos, and talk to other survivors. This book and others like it reveal that you are not alone!

I stated that when I first met Teri Dale, she was both a bundle of anxiety as well as a self-determined lightning bolt. I've since learned that this character quality makes her an ideal teacher and coach. She has learned to harness her anxiety into a tireless hunger to learn the truth. Once understood, she applies her knowledge with such tenacity that victory is all but guaranteed. She simply won't quit; losing is not an option. Maybe this is why we get along so well.

I pray that you use this book as a guide; use it to bring you hope. Use this book to assure that you are not alone. Reach out to Teri and I and others who are willing to help. Above all, reach out to God. Your cancer is no surprise to Him, and He wants nothing more than to bring you comfort through your pain.

Be Blessed,
Dr. Kevin Conners
Founder of Conners Clinic

INTRODUCTION

I remember the day I was told I had cancer. I remember what I was doing, what I was wearing, and where I was standing when that phone call came with the horrific news. I remember the instant nausea that set in. I remember the doctor's voice, and his abrupt tone that had no sense of compassion. I remember having to lean up against my kitchen counter, my head dropping, after hearing the words, "You have Hodgkin's Lymphoma."

All I heard was, I have cancer; all I heard was, I am going to suffer; all I heard was, I'm going to lose my hair; all I heard was, I'm going to be in terrible pain; all I heard was, I could possibly die. All I heard was, I'd be sick all of the time and that my quality of life was over. I had hundreds of thoughts cycle through my mind. None were positive. There was an awkward silence as I stood there in disbelief. My husband sat there quietly, staring at the ground, not saying a word. I could tell he was concerned and he didn't know what to say.

Amidst the shock of the moment was the disbelief that I could even get cancer. I have been a health and nutrition coach for over 20 years. I was active, I ate healthy, I exercised, I didn't use harmful substances, and there was no history of lymphoma in my family. I've helped thousands of clients prevent disease, get healthy, get off medications, lose weight, and "get their sexy back." … and BAM! … I get cancer? Seriously? How? Why? Now what?

I was in denial. You probably were, too, when you first learned about your diagnosis. I felt totally numb as I hung up the phone. I couldn't even cry. I was in shock and I didn't want to believe it. There had to be some mistake.

My husband, Mark, and I stood there in complete silence for at least two minutes, trying to really let it sink in. I'm not sure it *was* really sinking in. I was trying my hardest to think my way to a positive spin on the news, or how to make it go away, either with a solution or a reprieve: maybe it was a mistake? My husband didn't say a word. He was waiting for me to say something. I looked up at him, "I can't believe this. This can't be true, this feels like a nightmare. Mark, what are we going to do?" It wasn't until I said those words that the tears came. Mark grabbed me, gave me a hug, and said, "Everything is going to be fine. We'll figure it out."

I didn't want to hear everything was going to be fine. I didn't want to have to "figure it out." I just wanted it to go away. I didn't want to have cancer; I didn't want to deal with this. I can't have cancer. I just can't. I didn't want to accept it. I didn't want to believe it. It was the worst feeling and the most confusing moment I've ever experienced. It literally felt like I was just told I was going to die. Every time I think about this moment — write about it or share it with someone — I can't get through it without feeling a host of emotions and tearing up. It was so hard. No one will ever understand that feeling unless it happens to them.

I wrote this book for you, my dear friend. Why? Because I know what it feels like to be told the worst news of your life. I know what it feels like to feel helpless, out of control, and uncertain, scared and wondering what your next steps are. You are terrified about how you are going to be a mother while dealing with cancer. You are terrified about losing your hair and your health. You are fearful that your quality of life will be diminished by hospital stays and being sick in bed. You are worried you won't see your kid's graduation or wedding. You are worried about your finances. You are scared how cancer will affect your marriage. You are confused about what to do and where to go next. You are angry, then sad, then confused, then worried, then mad again.

In this book, I'll tell you about my decision to refuse chemo, and what I did instead to make space for my body (and God) to cure my lymphoma in only nine months. But equally important was my why. How could I fly in the face of popular wisdom and oncologists and go my own way?

It wasn't an easy decision, but it was a relatively simple one. How could I REFUSE chemo and radiation? Truly, how could I *not*? I mean, given who I am and everything I believe in, this had to be the direction I would choose. I am a functional diagnostic nutritionist, one who practices what she teaches. I have seen amazing turnarounds in my clients' health over the years, from diseases like obesity, type 2 diabetes, fibromyalgia, thyroid disorders, hormone imbalances, high cholesterol, heart disease, chronic fatigue syndrome, adrenal fatigue, anxiety, depression — the list goes on and on.

What it came down to for me was: How is cancer different than any other disease of the body? (Other than it's cancer, of course.) I have seen the power of my clients' shifts, and watched them heal from many diseases, some of them incredibly challenging. So deep down, I knew I had to roll up my sleeves, go against the mainstream, and learn about cancer and how it could be cured naturally. Scary? Yep. But I honestly wasn't willing to do it any other way, so it was full speed ahead.

I can truly understand your disbelief, anger, fear, and despair. I know the traditional cancer treatments available, and they are very bleak, daunting, and even harmful. Even though I was pretty clear on my choice of what I *wanted* to do, I wasn't clear on whether I *could* do it. Meaning, would I find a way to NOT do chemo and radiation? I talked to people who underwent chemo and radiation. I read their stories. I saw what they had to go through. I watched them deteriorate. I witnessed how the treatments killed them, literally. I did not want to live that way, suffering and in pain. I had some decisions to make.

My primary desire for you, in reading this book, is to understand that you have options other than chemo and radiation. But it's also very important for you to understand that YOU. HAVE. TIME. You do *not* need to rush, rush, rush into chemo and radiation right away. I didn't know what to do right away when I was first diagnosed. But what I did know was that I had spent all of my professional life learning about how the body can heal itself, and I was not going to let anyone push me into anything I wasn't 100% confident about and committed to doing. I knew I was facing a profound decision that would impact the rest of my life.

The wicked reality of cancer treatment is that mainstream therapies are pushed on the newly diagnosed very heavily and very fast. What's the reason for this big rush? Why do oncologists so adamantly want you in their system so quickly? Why won't they encourage you to look into holistic options or discuss alternative treatments with you? Why do they tell you that chemo and radiation are your only options? Why doesn't your oncologist talk to you about your diet? I can't wait to explain all of this to you. My hope is that it will empower you and bring you some peace of mind so that you can make the decision that is best for you.

This book is my true story of what I went through: the research, the conversations, the appointments, the confusion, the tears, the thoughts, and, of course, the solution. I am eager to share with you what I did in the hope that you will feel encouraged. I am devoted to you, my reader. I can't wait to share with you what many oncologists and doctors never will. They won't, because they can't. They *don't actually know.*

This is where you come in. When you increase your knowledge, that knowledge becomes power. And with this power comes your path to healing. Let's go!

*Please note that many of the chapters have actual, real-life client stories. I have changed the names and some of the details to protect their privacy, but the stories and incidents are true. I do not claim that this book will solve all of your health issues, but it's a start.

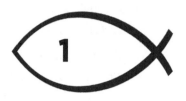

MY STORY

Health is a relationship between you and your body.

– Terri Guillemets

Mark and I were on our way up north to celebrate my parents' 50th wedding anniversary. I was really looking forward to spending the day with my entire family and visiting with friends and relatives, many of whom we hadn't seen in a long time. We were just a few miles from the church when I pulled down the visor to look in the mirror and check my lipstick and hair.

I noticed a lump on the right side of my neck. I immediately felt it, and it was hard. My immediate reaction was one of panic; I felt an instant rush of adrenaline and warmth fill my body. I looked in the mirror again … and then one more time. It was a pretty big lump. Why hadn't I noticed it before? My thoughts went right to the worst: a lump! Is it cancer? Then my thoughts veered away again. Nah... it can't be. I'm too healthy to get cancer. It has to be something else.

My parents' 50th wedding anniversary celebration, which was supposed to be a fun and joyous day, turned into a day of distraction and worry for me instead. I couldn't stop thinking about the lump in my neck — but I kept this to myself until the drive home.

As we made our way home from the church, I mentioned my finding to Mark. His reaction was a practical, "Well, go get it checked out." My reaction was immediate and intense: *No! I don't want to!* I decided it had to be just a swollen gland, and that thought managed to give me mental rest until we arrived home.

I went straight to the Internet and Googled "swollen gland." What I found wasn't very comforting, that's for sure. This led me to search, "Why do lymph nodes swell up?" and then on to "causes of swollen lymph nodes," "symptoms," "cancer," and "lymphoma." Ugh! I couldn't stand to consider this outcome. I decided just to keep an eye on the lump, and to ask one of my clients, an oncology physician's assistant, what she thought. (The one great thing about what I do, is I get to coach a lot of doctors, nurses, and people in the medical field. As you will learn later on in this book, they don't get any nutrition coaching in medical school, so they come to me to get help in this area.)

That next week, I asked my client what she thought. She looked at and felt my neck, and right away, I freaked out at the expression on her face.

She said, "Teri, you need to go get that checked out."

"Why?" I asked her. "I feel fine." Thinking back, I was just telling myself I felt fine. The truth was, I had a lot of fatigue and just generally did not feel my best. I think I had attributed it to hormonal shifts and stress.

Per her advice, I decided to see my primary physician and get some blood work done. I was also strongly encouraged to get a CAT scan, so I did — reluctantly. Frankly, I was scared to know what was going on.

I had so much blood drawn, I felt like I was making a donation. We checked everything. Out of all of the labs run, the only lab that came back anything less than normal was a low Vitamin D level, a not-uncommon finding among North Americans. But the CAT scan results were worrying. They showed I had many enlarged lymph nodes in the area of my neck on both sides, and the doctors suspected lymphoma. The next step would be a biopsy.

The entire time up to this point was a whirlwind of emotions. My blood work coming back all normal, was, at the time, a huge YAY! I didn't learn until later that more times than not, blood work can come back normal even in the later stages of cancer. But the CAT scan results were very unsettling.

I tend to be a worrier. So when I went in for the biopsy, it was a huge ordeal for me. The process itself was very simple, but the day leading up to it was not. Here's the deal: I am a very driven, type A, go-go-go, have-to-be-in-control type of person. I also had a lot of stress in my life at the time, and the diagnostic process didn't help. In the back of my mind, I understood that I potentially had cancer, and that was absolutely horrifying to me. It kept me awake at night, and it caused me to shut down many days with worry and concern. At this point, I had stopped doing any research, because it was just too overwhelming for me to think about. And honestly?

Deep down, I kept thinking, "God would not allow this to happen to me." I forced myself to believe that it was just a scare for me to get back on track with Him and my relationship, and a lesson that I need to slow down and work on my stress. I was not "accepting the realization" that it could be cancer very well at all.

On Wednesday, January 12th, I had a post-biopsy follow-up appointment with my ear,

nose, and throat doctor. Praise God! The biopsy came back negative for Hodgkin's Lymphoma!

Well, hold on a minute!

Me: "Doc, this is great news, right?"

Doc: "Well, Teri, biopsies are inconclusive and many times test out negative. I really think you should have surgery to remove the entire node."

Me: "What? I don't understand. Why would you have me do a biopsy if you knew that the results would be inconclusive?"

Doc: "This is just our normal process, we always biopsy first and then my suggestion is to surgically remove the actual node. When they remove the node, they actually cut it up into hundreds of pieces and look at it under a microscope, this way we will know for sure."

Me: "This makes no sense. Could it be an infection?"

Doc: "I really don't think so, but I will gladly give you antibiotics to try, and if that doesn't work, I strongly advise you to get it removed so we have a diagnosis. I wouldn't mess around with this too much longer."

At this point, I was not thinking I had lymphoma. I was trying to stay positive. I did try the antibiotics, although I usually resist taking them, because I was thinking, well, if it's an infection, then the node will go down.

The node didn't go down. After weeks of thinking about the pros and cons of having surgery to remove the node, I decided to go ahead. I was at the point where I was sick of worrying about it and not knowing for sure what was going on. Plus, visually, it was bothering me.

On Friday, March 4th, I went in for what was supposed to be a pretty simple procedure. But after surgery, I got really sick from the anesthesia and whatever other medications they had used for the procedure. I mean really, really sick. It was horrible. I was throwing up, got a migraine, had hot and cold spells, and I couldn't get out of bed for two and a half days.

The following Wednesday, I had my follow-up appointment with the doc/surgeon to go over the results of the pathology report, and also to make sure my incision was healing well.

Doc: "Well, I have good news and bad news."

Me: "Ok, let's hear the good news first."

Doc: "The pathology report came back negative."

Me: "Whoo hoo! See? I told you I didn't think I had cancer."

Doc: "Hold on, Teri. The bad news is that I suspect I removed the wrong gland."

(Silence as he reached over to take a peek at my neck.)

Doc: "The pathology report stated that the gland they dissected was a saliva gland, not the lymph node. We really need to verify this by you going and having another CAT scan today and then, if it is the case that the node is still in there, we should get you in for surgery immediately so that you don't build up scar tissue. It would be best to get in for surgery as soon as possible so that scar tissue doesn't start to form, which could cause nerve damage to your face and other complications."

Ok... so at this point, I am not going to continue on with the dialogue that ensued between Mark and the doctor. Mark was livid. While he expressed himself colorfully with a few choice words, I sat there in disbelief and complete horror. I went into full-on panic mode. I called my mom immediately and told her to call everyone she knew to pray for me. The thought of having another surgery almost did me in. I had a complete melt-down. Later that day, the CAT scan confirmed that the doctor had REMOVED THE WRONG FLIPPIN' GLAND IN MY NECK!! ARE YOU KIDDING ME RIGHT NOW!?

Surgery number two was exactly one week from my first. This one went much better this time. We made sure we had another doc in there to prevent further mistakes. The following Wednesday, at my follow-up appointment, the doctor said the pathology report from the University of Minnesota came back negative, but he wanted to send it off to the Mayo Clinic for a final analysis.

So at this point, as you can imagine, I was losing faith and confidence in the medical system. First, why did they tell me to do a biopsy if they knew they were going to suggest surgery anyway? Then they removed my saliva gland instead of my lymph node. Next, the biopsy came back negative, but the doc didn't trust the source so it had to go out for another opinion. The entire process was extremely agitating, confusing, and maddening.

Now, in hindsight, I wish I had slowed things down and done more research. But, like you, I'm sure, you trust your doctors, right? I mean, they are the professionals. They are supposed to be the ones trained to give you the best care, the best advice, and the best choices, right? Well, not when it comes to cancer. Cancer is truly an industry — and a money-making one at that. Yep, I said it — and I will back up this statement in Chapter 3.

One week later, on Friday, March 18th at 3:42 pm, we got the call. I remember nervously anticipating this call all week. I had just had a conversation with Mark an hour before telling him that I really didn't think I had cancer. I mean, two negative biopsies? What were the odds?

As I mentioned earlier in this book, the day I got the news is the most horrific memory of my adult life. Mark and I were standing in the kitchen chatting when the phone rang. We both stood there and listened to the doctor say, "The pathology report came back and you have Nodular Lymphocyte Predominate Hodgkin's Lymphoma. I will give you the name of an oncologist. I suggest you set up an appointment with her next week."

I couldn't move … I couldn't think … I couldn't cry. The only words in my head were, "I HAVE CANCER." This moment in time will always be fresh in my memory. The emotions that ran through my body were so horrifying. It's hard to even explain, it's like you are suddenly thrown into shocking contemplation of pain, suffering, and death. It's an instant change in your mind, and in your entire physiology. My heart starting pounding, I got hot, my stomach instantly got queasy, I felt lightheaded, I got weak — all this in just seconds.

After a few minutes of trying to gather my bearings and come to terms with what I was told, I went to my computer, and immediately started Googling "lymphoma." "What is lymphoma?" "How do you get lymphoma?" "Is lymphoma treatable?" What I discovered was daunting, discouraging, and alarming. I could hardly read the words on the computer through my tears. Were chemo and radiation the only solutions for treatment? Could they actually even cure the cancer? All I was seeing and reading was that these two treatments were the only treatments offered at cancer clinics.

Then I started reading up on what chemotherapy actually is and what it does … ummmm … I was not willing to put poison in my body. I mean, seriously, I had served many years in the health coaching industry, and suddenly, at 49 years old, I was sitting there facing what I felt was a death sentence. I thought, "God? Why are you punishing me this way? What have I done to deserve cancer?" Not only was I facing what I thought were my only options, chemo and radiation, but it also looked like I would have to do both as the required treatment. This was too much for me to handle. I had to close my computer and not deal with this anymore. Needless to say, I was full of despair, anguish, and questions.

I didn't sleep well at all. I got up early the next morning and was tempted to call one of my staff members to see if they would fill in for me so I wouldn't have to go in and face my clients. What in the world are they going to think? I was feeling like a hypocrite. I was feeling embarrassed. To my clients, I am their teacher and coach, someone they look up to. Someone who educates them about all the aspects of living a well-balanced and healthy lifestyle, who preaches health and fitness — and I end up with cancer. I was so mad. So, so mad. "How can I lead and teach these ladies," I thought, "if I have cancer?"

Looking back, I sure beat myself up, didn't I? I am sure you are also beating yourself up. When we get news of this magnitude, we react in so many different ways, and frequently that first reaction is equal parts denial and self-blame. It's so horrifying that it's tempting to do something — anything! — but what I learned is that you must dig deep. You must *slow* down and not make decisions when you are in a state of panic, fear, anger, or confusion. Take your time reading this book, as well as others, so that you can fuel yourself with information and get your power back. You will be more equipped to fight when you are calmer, more educated, and less overwhelmed.

Back then, though, I didn't know any of this yet. I was sure I had to make some sort of decision almost immediately, and I was equally sure that I couldn't tell my clients I had cancer. A perfect recipe for complete panic. I didn't want to go in to my gym that next morning with this weight on my shoulders, but I had to. When I got there, I tried my best to hold it together, taught my cardio kickboxing class, put on a fake smile and my "nothing is wrong" disguise, and then hurried off to my office to have a meltdown.

It was so tough. I wanted to tell them, but I couldn't. I was embarrassed, scared, and worried. I was their leader. They couldn't see me as weak. I worried that I would lose my business. If I was going to be sick from the chemo and radiation, how would I teach my classes? How could I run a business if I was sick all of the time? How would I be able to coach my clients? How would I be able to speak in public and give presentations on health and wellness when I didn't look healthy and well?

My thoughts scrambled on. I didn't want to lose my hair. My maintaining a healthy, fit appearance was important to what I did for a living — how was this going to work? I didn't want anyone seeing me sick. I didn't want to put poison in my body. I didn't want to look emaciated. Even though I was strongly opposed to doing chemo, I wasn't yet convinced that I wouldn't have to. I mean, I hadn't yet learned of any holistic alternatives, and I was terrified that chemo might be my only option. Tears … floods of tears … the pity party was next.

My pity party lasted a day. I moped, cried, felt sorry for myself, and questioned God. I was very disappointed and angry. I can't ever remember feeling as dejected, down, scared, mad, frustrated, worried, and confused all at the same time. It was the ickiest process I have ever had to face. I kept trying to figure out what the lesson was, if there was one. Why, God? I asked Him to reveal to me what He was doing. I mean, two surgeries? *Two* negative biopsies? What was the point?

It felt too big for me to deal with. "I can't do it," I thought. "I don't want to try. I give up. I quit." I wanted to just hide. I tried to think of the ways I could get out of facing my clients and deal with my cancer in my own private way. It was all so overwhelming to me. I truly felt like giving up. Quitting everything. I mean, *everything*.

Whoa. Wait.

With these thoughts rampant upon me, something sparked. I thought, "Stop it, Teri. You have to stop thinking like this. Turn it around, now." I thought about what I knew about myself. I knew I was not a quitter. I was a fighter. I was very smart. I had never given up before when things had been hard. Even though this was definitely the most serious and difficult challenge I'd had in my life, I'd had other challenges and I got through them. I had clients all around me who I'd helped regain their health. What made this situation any different? Other than it's me, not a client, and it's my cancer, not someone else's illness?

This was my defining moment. My fighter spirit rekindled, I received this power shot of energy, and all of a sudden, my thoughts became those of a conqueror, not a victim. I do believe it was God turning my thinking around. He gave me the spiritual guidance (intuition) that I needed at that moment to start figuring out another path to heal my body and make the decision to REFUSE chemo. I decided to take back my power instead of letting the doctors have it. Enough! Enough of the "I don't know what to do, I can't deal with this" mentality. I just needed to follow what I already knew, which was that, given the right things, the body can heal itself. I would be my own client.

In fact, I'd done just this a dozen years earlier, when I was diagnosed with adrenal fatigue, a condition most commonly associated with intense or prolonged stress. I was able to reverse it with nutrition, lifestyle, supplements, and holistic options, just as I helped my clients with their health issues.

I reminded myself that going through adrenal fatigue had been very challenging, while not as serious as cancer. I came to the realization that I could fight cancer, just like I'd chosen to fight adrenal fatigue. I had been through tough times before, and I had complete faith in myself to fight for my health once again, and the outcome would be the same: victory and healing! I just had to figure out the direction to heal cancer just like I'd had to figure out the direction to heal adrenal fatigue.

This instantly flipped the switch on my thoughts, and I felt a surge of power to fight, learn, prove my oncologist wrong, and prove to the world that cancer could be cured with holistic options. Meditating on this gave me courage. It gave me a goal, and it gave me hope. I had decided. *This* was the moment that I made the decision to REFUSE chemo, heal my cancer, take control of the situation, and let God totally direct my path to my healing.

Giving God the reins was a huge relief, and it was also exactly the right thing for me to do. Have you ever been in a situation where you felt crippled by your circumstance, but once you figured out a plan or a way to go about dealing with it, you felt empowered? This is what taking back your power does. Having the confidence to fight, trust your instincts, and make a decision that coincides with your strong beliefs and convictions no matter what others think — *this* is what gives you the strength and momentum to move forward. My opinion is that taking back your power is the single most important step in starting your healing journey.

It was also at this moment that I realized that my poor body was sick for a reason. I knew I simply had to learn and understand why. I just had to think of myself as my own client. If someone came to me with a condition or disease, what would I tell them? I have always been motivated to find the cause of a particular ailment or health issue, not just treat the symptom. My body has cancer. Cancer is the symptom … the symptom of something. But what? Armed with what I knew about the body and buoyed by how many times I'd seen my clients reverse many of their diseases, I was on a mission to be my own health advocate and figure it out.

After this huge mental switch, I started to feel encouraged. I thought about feeling good again. I envisioned my body being healed. I thought about how much I would be learning; about how amazing it would be to be able to heal my body of cancer without all of the horrible side effects that traditional treatments bring. I thought about being able to continue to coach my clients and work while healing my body. I thought about being able to exercise and teach classes; about still being able to give presentations with vigor and energy. I thought about still being able to get my hair done. I thought about being able to go out with friends and family. I even thought about the bigger picture … like, maybe someday I will be able to help others through this process. (Yes!)

I didn't want to look like a cancer patient. I wanted people to look at me and have no clue that I was fighting cancer. Yes, this lit a fire in me. It got me even more energized and focused on what I needed to do next. I longed for the day that I could say, my PET scan is *clean*. I no longer have cancer. I was so going to do this … I needed to do this. I sat down and prayed. With my heavenly Father's help, guidance, discernment, and direction, I knew this was the path He was leading me on. Here is my actual prayer that I copied from my journal.

> *Dear Lord — I am confident that you are almighty God and you will work wonders on my behalf. I ask you to fight for me and bring me through to victory. I know you are with me and I ask you to guide my path.… Show me, reveal to me how you want me to deal with this situation. I have no idea where to start. I TRUST YOU! I LOVE YOU! I WORSHIP YOU.… I NEED YOU!! Make my decisions so very clear to me and reveal to me your guiding presence of the Holy Spirit. AMEN.*

Wouldn't it be awesome if you had clarity, discernment, confidence, and knowledge? You must get your power back if you are going to fight this. This is a battle, not only with yourself but with everyone around you. I want to help you so that you don't feel all alone, as I did. I wish I'd had someone to talk to, to give me advice and help me and guide me. Someone to discuss options with, someone who'd also chosen to reject chemo and radiation.

This is one of the reasons why I created the REFUSED Solution, to give you the knowledge, encouragement, and support I wish I'd had back then. It's based on my own experience figuring out how to build my immune system, find the imbalance going on, and heal my body without chemo or radiation. My life was at stake, so I dug deep. I compiled my years of nutrition expertise, combined all the new research studies, case studies, interviews, and scientific reports I'd studied, and put it in a program that cured my cancer.

The REFUSED Solution will guide you through this entire process. After your diagnosis, you have time! You really do, no matter what you are told. Let me say that again, because it is so important that you understand this. *You have time after you are diagnosed.* Time to take a few weeks, to take it all in, to think about things, and to come up with your game plan. When I went through my own steps, I felt power, relief, motivation, and healing. This gave me momentum and courage. It was the best decision I ever made.

Let me show you how to do it. Here is the 7-Step REFUSED Solution:

R — Research

E — Environmental Toxins

F — Food

U — Unite with God

S — Supplements

E — Eliminating Stress

D — Detox

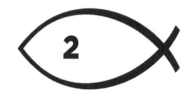

FACING YOUR FEAR

ref·use

rə ˈfyōoz/

verb: indicate or show that one is not willing to do something.

"Teri, wake up, can you hear me?"

As I woke up, I thought, "Oh, yay, I'm alive and I survived surgery!" But my second thought was about how bad I felt. My head was pounding. I was nauseated and thought I might throw up. Even after two hours post-op at the surgery center, I still wanted to do nothing but lie down with an ice pack on my head. I was soooo sick. I barely remember the drive home from the hospital. As soon as I got home, I immediately began throwing up. Like, every 30 minutes. All night long. In between bouts of vomiting, my head hurt so bad that I couldn't rest.

The next morning, I was still in the same shape — throwing up, head pounding, neck throbbing — and all I could think of was, "If this is how I feel with just anesthesia, I can't even imagine how sick I'll be with chemo and radiation." My body was simply not used to having junk put in it. I couldn't even remember the last time I took an ibuprofen, or cold medication, or aspirin, or anything that was not a vitamin or supplement. Was this a glimpse of what I would be dealing with for the rest of my life?

Like you, I looked up side effects of chemo: fatigue, hair loss, nausea, vomiting, constipation, digestion issues, diarrhea, sore tongue, repeated infections, appetite changes, migraines, infections, lightheadedness, pale skin, difficulty thinking, weakness, anxiety, depression, hormonal fluctuations, infertility, bone marrow suppression, neuropathy, joint pain, edema, bladder irritation, kidney damage, increased risk of osteoporosis, bone fractures, and other cancers. Wait, *and other cancers*?

Then I looked up the side effects of radiation: skin problems, dryness, itching, blistering and peeling, fatigue, dry mouth, gum sores, difficulty swallowing, stiffness in the jaw, nausea, swelling, shortness of breath, stiffness, cough, fever … the list goes on, depending on where on your body you have the radiation.

Aren't these side effects horrifying? Like me, you probably don't want to accept a lifetime of being sick, in pain, suffering, or bedridden. You don't want to lose your hair, look sick, and, more than likely, be unable to maintain the quality of life that you so want.

I had a small taste of the pain and suffering after anesthesia, and that was enough for me. As a long time fitness expert and functional diagnostic nutrition coach, putting poison and radiation in my body didn't make sense to me. I found it hard to believe that I would have to get sicker in order to get better. I reminded myself of three core things:

1) I had to be my own client. I had to coach myself the same way I would have coached any one of my clients who'd come to me with this problem.

2) I was not and am not a quitter. I am a fighter, and I don't give up.

3) My office was full of case studies featuring many clients I'd helped with numerous health conditions, and with my help, they'd been able to reverse their disease.

So the answer is, you *don't* have to get sick before you get better. I didn't just hypothesize this. I proved it. I proved that you can heal your body of cancer without radiation or chemotherapy, because I did it for myself. Once I was healed, I identified the seven steps I used to cure myself and created the REFUSED Solution. These seven steps healed my body of Stage II Nodular lymphocyte-predominant Hodgkin's lymphoma (nLPHL) in nine months.

If you thoroughly understand and really take the time to apply these steps, I am convinced you will be able to heal your body. Now, I want to emphasize this: I am not a doctor. But I am a woman who has made it her life mission to help others as a functional diagnostic nutritionist (FDN) and coach. I cannot promise or guarantee that you will be cured or healed, but the seven steps I created and followed worked for me.

Before I explain what the REFUSED Solution entails, you first need to understand what lymphoma is. Lymphoma is a cancer of the lymph nodes. It affects the white blood cells (called lymphocytes) of the immune system. These cells are in the lymph nodes, spleen, thymus, bone marrow, and other parts of body. There are two types of lymphoma: non-Hodgkin's and Hodgkin's. Both originate in the lymphatic system, but the main difference is in the specific lymphocyte each involves. Lymphoma is staged based on the extent of the lymphoma as well as where in the body you have enlarged nodes, for example, neck, chest, abdomen, and/or pelvis.

Stage I

The cancer is found only in a single region or organ, usually one lymph node and the surrounding area.

Stage II

The cancer is found in two or more lymph node regions on the same side of the diaphragm, either above or below it.

Stage III

The cancer is found in lymph nodes on both sides of the diaphragm.

Stage IV

The cancer has spread to one or more tissues or organs outside the lymph system (e.g., liver, lungs, bones), and may be in lymph nodes near or far from those organs.

Also, in addition to the numerical staging component, the letters A, B, E, and S are used to help describe the cancer. The letters A and B indicate the presence or absence of certain symptoms. The letters E and S refer to the spread of the disease beyond the lymph nodes.

A & B

The letter B indicates the presence of one or more of the following symptoms: drenching night sweats, fever, or unexplained weight loss. The letter A is used if there is no evidence of B symptoms.

E & S

The letter E indicates the disease affects extranodal tissues or organs (areas outside of the lymph system). The letter S is used if the disease has spread to the spleen. From what my oncologist said and from all the reading I did on Hodgkin's and non-Hodgkin's lymphoma, it is said to have a very high success rate with chemo and radiation working to kill the cancer and shrink the tumors. So in my mind, I immediately thought, well, if conventional treatment is supposed to work but it's essentially poison — we know chemo kills our immune system function and our healthy cells and damages the entire body long-term — then why wouldn't putting natural treatments in your body work even better? Plus, natural treatments have *no* harmful side effects. Almost everyone I've talked to who has done chemo and radiation had long-lasting, unpleasant side effects, and in many cases, the cancer came back anyway. So it made sense to me that if, instead of destroying my immune system, I could build it up so it could do its job (which, among other things, is to kill and fight cancer), then why would I even want to willingly put poison in my body and risk the immune system devastation and other harmful side effects?

The reason most people quickly rush to chemo and radiation is because they are scared and being pushed heavily by their oncologists to do so. They are being pressured by their family and friends, who think they're crazy for not undergoing conventional treatments.

I get it, I really do. But I am hoping that after reading this book, you will learn that you have time to research your options, get your power back, and make a decision that you feel peaceful about. What I learned is that when we don't do our due diligence or find our own truth, we make decisions based on fear and inaccurate information. I am here to help you with this confusion.

Here's the deal. It doesn't matter what kind of cancer you have. If you have any kind of cancer, the cells in your body have, for some reason, grown out of control, likely because they have been damaged by a plethora of things like carcinogens and toxins. Your immune system simply isn't working properly to kill the unhealthy and damaged cells.

> *"Cancer is a disease of the entire body, not just a body part — without exception. So if you have a doctor that gets on the offensive and just attacks the tumor, or treats only the area of your body with cancer (surgery, radiation), then he/ she is ignoring the fact that the cancer is a result of sickness in your entire body, and that it isn't just the tumor that needs to be treated, but ALL OF YOU!"*
>
> – Leigh Erin Connealy, MD, *The Cancer Revolution*

This is the key. You must treat the entire body and fix the entire system — and *that* requires a total lifestyle change. When a client comes to me with a health problem, the first thing I do is seek to understand their entire situation and figure out the underlying cause of the issue. I was trained to be a health detective, to learn what is out of balance in the body to cause the symptom, and then fix that imbalance. This is not the allopathic medical model, which instead identifies the symptom and then finds a drug to alleviate that symptom. That's totally backwards.

You can't treat just one area of the body and then expect the disease, any disease, to permanently go away. Cancer is no different. My client Cindy is a perfect case in point. Cindy was diagnosed with colon cancer and had surgery to remove some of her colon and some enlarged nodes. She didn't want to do chemo and radiation, but she wasn't sure where to start, so she hired me. As she was healing from surgery, I had her start the REFUSED Solution I'll be sharing with you in upcoming chapters.

She had not even been staged yet when she went back to her oncologist three weeks later. He told her that the tumors they'd removed were cancerous, but the nodes they'd removed were not. It looked like the cancer was isolated in the tumors. Her PET scan was clean, and so was her bone marrow, which meant that she had no other cancerous tumors anywhere in her body. Great news, right? But wait: her oncologist told her she had to start chemo and radiation right away to make sure the cancer didn't come back. You know, just as a preventative. What the what?! Clean scan, clean bone marrow, clean blood work ... and he wants to put her on chemo and poison in her body "just because"?

This is my whole point. They push treatments and freak you out without giving you any info on what any of these results actually mean. Cindy is not doing chemo and radiation. She has been educated now and is so happy and relieved. She got her power back. She is taking control of her situation. She is learning for herself. By hiring me, she was able to avail herself of the lessons I learned from my hard-won experience and of tons of resources, advice, and help. She was able to make her own decision to not do chemo, and feel good about that choice. She has found that working with someone to help her sort out all the confusion was helpful, and that it also has given her the tools to be able to communicate her decision better with her family.

Cindy is working her way through the REFUSED Solution. Because Cindy had a cancerous tumor in her body, we know she has CTCs (I will be explaining in detail later what these are) circulating around in her blood, so we want to make sure to build up her immune system so it's able to kill the CTCs and not create new tumors. She is working on healing her entire body. Can you see how, if she would have chosen chemo, it would have not fixed her imbalance and potentially made things worse?

The REFUSED Solution

I want to help you get your power back so you feel confident in making a decision to refuse chemo. I understand the fear you have and the pressure you are getting from everyone around you. The REFUSED Solution contains your first steps to try, and they are extremely important for you to understand before making this life and death decision. I want to be right next to you, coaching and helping you with every step. This is my promise to you.

R: Research

In order to be confident in your decision, you *must* be willing to dig in and not only learn about your specific kind of cancer, but also about all your treatment options. Most people never get past reading about the chemo and radiation protocols, and then they are so scared and frightened that they immediately panic, defer to their doctors (who are human, by the way, and do make mistakes), and don't do their due diligence and learn about both ways of treating their cancer. There are *two* kinds of treatment: chemo and radiation (called allopathic treatment), and alternative/holistic treatment. You *have-have-have* to learn about both: what they are, how they work, and the implications of each.

This is key to your healing, your peace of mind, and your taking your power back. Too many give all their power to their doctors instead of being their own health advocates. Use your doctor to ask informed questions so you can make a better decision. When I give you a sneak peek inside the cancer industry, you will start to see what you are *not* being told. Chances are, you don't even know about your holistic options — or don't know what they even consist of, let alone if they even work. You've been told that a combination of chemo and radiation is your only option, and if you don't do it, you will either get worse or die. I am here to tell you otherwise. There is a whole other world, a world that your oncologist doesn't understand or know anything about. This is what you have to understand before choosing any treatment plan. Know your options. Hold tight! Info is on its way.

E: Environment

How much do you know about your environment and the effect it has on your health — specifically in developing cancer? Many people believe we are somehow protected from environmental harm: Why would the government allow us to be in danger? The sad reality is that we live in a very toxic world, and the manufacturing industry is a huge part of this issue. There are many environmental factors that are making us sick. Our bodies get overloaded, and that toxic overload increases our risk of cancer. What caused your cancer? If I knew this answer, I'd be a millionaire 100 times over. The truth is, we have a lot of updated research that reveals the truth: that specific hazardous chemicals impact the growth of cancer and suppression of your immune system. Some major risk factors of developing cancer are in our environment. These are things that you are exposed to every day. Some environmental exposures are impossible to avoid, like the air we breathe, the products we use, and the contaminated soil in which we plant our food. There are more, but understanding some of the major environmental risk factors will help you become more aware of your surroundings so that you can remove some of these environmental toxins from your life.

F: Food

This is my absolute favorite step! I enjoy talking about nutrition, and I am constantly learning how much it impacts our health and rids our bodies of disease. I love teaching my clients how food is their medicine — in fact, try to find anything in nature that is *not* medicine. The issue, in this day and age, is that most Americans eat processed food, food that has been heavily manufactured, all the healthy nutrients and enzymes removed and toxic chemicals added in that boost flavor, induce cravings, and keep us sick. I have always believed that what you put in your body is a reflection of your health. Back in 2006 when I learned I had adrenal fatigue, the only things that worked to reverse my condition were changing my diet and managing my stress levels. When you can understand how vital nutrition is to your health and healing, you will make the effort to eat healthy. Sadly, most people wait until they get sick before they decide to make dietary changes that improve health.

When I got diagnosed with cancer, I had to give nutrition a try first. There was just way too much evidence of reversal of disease attributed to the use of good nutrition strategies for me to ignore. Every bite you put in your mouth is either going to benefit your health — or not.

When you went to your oncologist or doctor and asked them about what you should be eating, what did they say? I bet I can guess. I have seen the menus they give out to their hospitalized cancer patients. It's mind-blowing. Here's what I do know, because I've asked oncologists and physicians: in med school, they get one day of nutrition classes (sometime less) in eight years of study. They do not understand or know about how food can impact your health. That is not what they are taught. They are heavily influenced in med school to use medications and procedures to alleviate or eliminate symptoms. They are not taught how to use nutrition as a form of natural medicine. This is a fact!

You are either eating to live or living to eat. If you are living to eat, then you are putting processed food, toxins, and chemicals in your body that will eventually lead you to poor health (which is one of the reasons you have cancer). Maybe you are living to eat because you have never been taught about nutrition, or maybe it's because you do not have an awareness about it but now are forced to learn about it. However, if you are eating to live, you are selecting nutrition that will nourish and energize your body. Every bite you take is then promoting your health instead of promoting disease.

In order to heal your cancer, you have to make radical changes in your diet. There is just no question about it. The good news is this: Once you start giving your body what it needs to fight the cancer, you will feel the best you ever have. Not only did I feel amazing and still do, but everyone that I talked to, interviewed, and helped all had this one common denominator: They felt amazing. Great energy, no debilitating symptoms, and no adverse reactions like with chemo and radiation. This in itself was one of my main motivators to learn even more about nutrition. I will take you through all of this.

U: Unite with God

Oh my dear friend, I can say with all honesty that this step, for me, was the most important of all. Cancer forced me to step out in faith and reconnect with God. I have to share my heart with you very deeply and intimately about this step. If it wasn't for my relationship with God and His leading me during this very stressful time, I would *not* be writing to you today. It is because of my cancer that I know God in a more intimate way. But when I was first diagnosed, I was mad, I was confused, I didn't understand why I had to get cancer.... I am sure you are feeling this exact same way. I want to share with you how God revealed these steps to me, how he changed my heart, how he molded me, how he taught me, and how he healed me. In my opinion, this is going to be the most important step for you to take seriously and try to implement in your life.

I am going to get intimate with you and share my deepest thoughts. I only am doing this because I hope it helps you. There were days when I felt so alone, discouraged, and sad. There were days when my faith was tested. But I knew that God was there, and He showed up time and time again. I want you to feel encouraged. I want you to have peace during this horrific time. I want you to have what I did, which was peace and direction. With God's help, you, too, can have this. God wants you to seek and understand Him and His will for your life. If you do that, He will lead you, direct you, and give you the answers you need. Until I decided to give my situation to God, I had despair, fear, and doubt. I had to trust His leading and study His word to receive encouragement and discernment. I also prayed daily for wisdom and healing.

The Bible is like your life manual. There is not any problem you have that the Bible doesn't have an answer for. You, too, will have answers. I want to help you. My hope is that you will read, reread and take this step to heart. It will be the most important one of them all.

S: Supplements

Did you know that supplements are food? Here's the deal. Medications are substances used for medical treatment. They are synthetic particles made to treat, not cure. Most medications have side effects. The medication might relieve a symptom, but more times than not, a new symptom will also appear. Eventually, it will lead to taking more medications. It's a vicious cycle. Although some dietary supplements are misrepresented and mislabeled, most are intended to provide nutrients that may otherwise be lacking in the human diet. Nutrients such as minerals, vitamins, etc. are best if derived from food sources, but sometimes we need to get additional nutrients into our bodies that we lack in our food supply.

I *love* supplements. Now, that doesn't mean I am a supplement pusher. In fact, I am of the opinion that your body only needs what it needs. You don't need an exorbitant amount of supplements. Most people take them just to take them, or they read an article making unrealistic claims, or they hear from a buddy that they should try such and such supplement. They spend way too much money on supplements that they don't need. Even though supplements are much safer then medications in the way they are absorbed and utilized in the body, they can still be dangerous if taken wrongly or when not needed. The entire point is to educate you on how you can use supplements in place of medications to heal. I will explain to you the benefits of the supplements I used to heal my cancer.

E: Eliminating Stress

Stressed out, overwhelmed, frustrated, exhausted, burned out, and discontent. These terms all described me before I was diagnosed with cancer. There were not enough hours in the day to get things done I needed to get done. Finances were tight, my work load was high, tough decisions had to be made, and I was on pure overload anxiety. I was also dealing with some relationship issues that brought on a huge plethora of stressful emotions. There is a link between stress and cancer. Stress impacts physiological processes in your body. It can cause certain hormones to be released that slow down parts of your immune system. Disease feeds off stress. This is not good when you are trying to fight cancer. If you don't deal with the stress in your life, it will greatly affect everything you try to do to heal your cancer. When you have chronic stress, whether mental/emotional, physical/biomechanical, or mostly just physiological, the negative impact on your ability to heal your cancer is significant. There are research studies that prove chronic or long-term stress impairs and suppresses your immune system. Your immune system is what *kills* cancer. We have to do all we can to build up our immune systems so they can heal us, and stress is a major problem when you are trying to reverse disease. So let's really get a handle on our stress levels, understand what stress does, determine what kind of stressors you have in play, and figure out a plan to reduce them.

D: Detox

When I say the word "detox," do you really understand what this even means? Many people think detoxing is about doing a series of colonics, or undertaking a 30-day starvation program where you can only drink liquids and take supplements. I've never done a colonic, nor have I ever starved myself by drinking only liquids and consuming supplements. I'm not saying colonics are bad; some cancer patients are so sick and constipated that they can't eliminate the waste that is rotting in their colons. In those cases, yes, colonics would be recommended. When you have cancer, your body is acidic. You must be able to eliminate those toxins every single day. We must make sure our detox pathways are available and working as well as make sure we are not continuing to bombard our body with chemicals inwardly and outwardly.

The issue is that we are exposed to toxins everywhere we look: our environment, food, water, products we use on our bodies (lotions, soaps, perfumes), products we use in our households (cleaners, detergents), and medications. We must learn where we are getting those toxins, what these toxins are, and how they impact our health. Once we understand this, then the next step is to eliminate certain products and chemicals from our grocery lists. Then we *must* get rid of the buildup of toxins in our bodies. When toxins enter your body, you become very acidic, which means that every organ in your body becomes a breeding ground for cancer. There are numerous ways to detox. Some are very fun, enjoyable, and relaxing — and others not. Just sayin'. We will go into detail about what you need to do to start detoxing on a daily basis, and talk about detox methods you can start immediately.

So now, let's dig into each step in detail so you can educate yourself, get your power back, and make the decision that will be best for you. First step: R (Research).

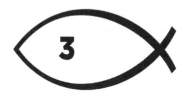

R — RESEARCH

*"After $ 600 billion spent on cancer research,
cancer remains un-cured."*

– Dr. Peter Glidden

After my cancer diagnosis, I waited a week before meeting with my oncologist. I wanted to gather information and learn as much as I could before I met with her. I had decided I was going to go holistic, but I thought maybe I could pick her brain and see what she knew about any alternative treatments. Quite honestly, after I made my decision to not do chemo and radiation, I really didn't even want to go and visit with her. I had so much anxiety about it, but I was getting pressure from my parents to at least go and hear what she had to say. I acquiesced and decided, ok, I'll go, but I am going to audio record the entire conversation and ask her a million questions. I thought I would probably learn something.

The day before my appointment with the oncologist, I called her office and left a message saying that I really needed to have a conversation with her before our meeting. When she called me back, I told her that I had already decided to go with alternative holistic options and asked her if she would be open to still meeting with me and supporting that decision. I told her that if she was not willing to support this decision, I would cancel our appointment. She said she would be willing to hear what I had in mind, but she also said that I was too young to be messing around with treatments that were not scientifically proven to be beneficial or work. She said that she would be very open, but would also go over what her treatment plan would be for me and that I should be open to listening to that.

What this oncologist didn't know was that my husband and I had already spent hours — I'm talking *hours* — reading books and articles about alternative treatments. We watched *The Truth About Cancer,* a phenomenal video series that covers all aspects of the cancer industry as well as interviews with dozens of doctors, scientists, and patients that have had proven success in healing cancer with alternative treatments. I love to research and learn. I have been doing this my entire career. When I had adrenal fatigue, I had to go against standard treatment, because at that time, there were not a lot of options out there for holistic treatments. I had to research and use my expertise to reverse my AF, and I did. So, cancer for me was no different. I had to study, research, educate myself, take classes, and talk to others to understand as much as I could about cancer, in order to take the steps I needed to heal myself. I was ready and equipped to share with the oncologist what I was learning.

But after hanging up the phone, I had so much trepidation about meeting with her. I had already made up my mind that I was going to give alternative methods a try, and I didn't want to feel like I was being pressured, forced, or scared into doing chemo and radiation. My gut was telling me that she would try to convince me to do things her way. I didn't want to hear about how she would treat me, I really didn't. I didn't want her to burst my confidence about the decision I had already made, and I was afraid that might happen. But my family insisted I go. And so, to appease them, I did.

As I walked down the hallway toward the oncologist's office, my stomach was in a knot. I was so uneasy about this appointment. I opened the door to the oncology office and … OH MY WORD!

As I walked in, I saw, immediately to my right, a line of patients receiving chemo. They all looked extremely sick. One woman was vomiting; most of them were wearing bandanas, or bald. Each one had a blanket covering their legs and feet, and they looked absolutely miserable.

I looked over to my left, into the waiting area. I saw men with walkers, women with wigs, many more bald women and men. There was not one person smiling in the entire place, not to mention the place smelled. Even the receptionists at the counter looked grumpy and didn't even acknowledge us when we walked in. Then I see, sitting on the counter top, a huge bowl of candy. (Don't they know that sugar is a cancer feeder?) I was and looked like the healthiest person there.

> Me, loudly, tears welling up in my eyes: "I can't. I just can't do this."

I quickly walked out into the hallway. By the time I got out there, I was bawling.

Mom, rushing out behind me: "Teri honey, it's going to be ok."

Me: "Mom, I can't, I really can't. This is like a nightmare. Look at this place. Everyone is so sick. Did you see those people in there getting chemo? Why would they have them right in open sight for everyone to see? I don't want to be exposed to this negative place. I don't want to be here."

Mom: "Why don't you just let me, Mark, and your dad go in and talk to the oncologist? You can just stay out here and wait and not even go in. Would that make you feel better?"

I was crying too hard to talk. A few moments later, Mark came out to see me.

Mark: "Teri, let's just go. We don't need to be here. I certainly don't need to talk with her. We've already made our decision, I am totally fine with leaving."

LONG PAUSE.

I could tell my mom was not very happy about the idea of us leaving. I understand her resistance to me choosing holistic treatment. She was scared for me. She wanted me well. But no one knew or knows what Mark and I had been starting to learn. We had only just begun our research and findings, and it was mind blowing what we were discovering.

If I knew I was going holistic and I was confident in my decision, then why was I so upset and why didn't I want to go visit with the oncologist? Well, I'm human. I was afraid. I was afraid of her telling me that I would be stupid to try something other than chemo. I was certain she would tell me holistic would not work. I was still emotional and vulnerable. I was not wanting anyone or anything to detour me from my mission of getting well, using the methods that I knew would work. I had such a strong intuition and message to *not* do chemo, and I didn't want to have doubt. I wanted to move forward with my plan.

> Mom: "Teri, you just stay out here, we will go in and talk with her."

> Me: "OK, that is what I want to do. I will be out here."

Half an hour went by, and my parents and Mark were still not called in to see the oncologist. After praying in the hallway, God calming me down, I decided I would go in and talk to her, too. After waiting for an entire hour, we were called in.

I will say this: my oncologist was actually very nice. She didn't come out and say, "You should do chemo and radiation or you're going to die," but I could sense that she was not comfortable about my plan to go holistic. She did try to answer every question I had. Most of my questions though, were questions she couldn't answer because she didn't know, which was alarming and baffling to me.

> Me: "So, doc, how would you treat me? After seeing my scans and knowing the type of lymphoma I have, what would be your next steps?"

Doc: "Well, I would weigh you, then I would look at the treatment most commonly used for Nodular lymphocyte-predominant Hodgkin's lymphoma and we would start you with chemo first to see how your body responds, and then add in radiation."

Me: "That's it? No other options that are less damaging?"

Doc: "What do you mean, 'damaging'? The good news, Teri, is that chemo and radiation for lymphoma have a very high success rate of remission. I have seen many of my patients have great luck with this treatment."

Me: "I don't want remission, I want to be cured. How many of those patients are still alive or have no more cancer, and how many have had their cancer come back or spread to other organs after their chemo treatments?"

Doc: (Long pause) "I can't answer that specifically. There is some risk of it not working and the cancer spreading, but of any of the cancers, chemo has been fairly successful with lymphoma."

Me: "Do you have any recommendations for nutritional supplements that would help with healing my cancer? Also, intravenous vitamin C therapy, do you offer that?"

Doc: 'Honestly, Teri, I cannot give you any recommendations on supplements. I could lose my medical license if I suggest something that is not a part of our standard cancer protocol. As far as vitamin C therapy, there has been some talk about the possibility of using this in the future, but at this time, we do not offer it as a part of our treatment plan."

(Just for your own info, intravenous vitamin C therapy is a high dose of vitamin C that is injected in your body to target and eradicate cancer cells that are lurking in the body. It must be administered by a trained physician, but is very safe and well-tolerated.)

Me: "Do you do chemo sensitivity testing?"

Doc: "What's that?"

Me: "It's where you draw blood and test different chemotherapy drugs to see if the chemo will even work in my body. Because as you know, many chemotherapy treatments don't even work on certain individuals based on their DNA. You do know this, right?"

Doc: "We do not do chemo sensitivity testing."

Me: "Do you offer IPT therapy? "

Doc: "Again, I am not aware of this treatment."

Me: "Well, Doc, it actually is a very low-dose chemo treatment that uses insulin with the chemotherapy to fool cancer cells. It allows a very low dose of chemo, which is less toxic and selectively hits cancer cells versus just blasting the whole body with chemo."

Doc: "Hmmm, that sounds interesting, what's it called again? I will have to read up on that." (She didn't have knowledge of any of the holistic cancer treatments that I asked her about. I was miffed. I knew more than she did, which seemed crazy.)

Me: "So, you are telling me that you would weigh me, look in a treatment book, start me on chemo next week, have me go look at wigs, and then, after 10 treatments, you would start radiation."

Doc: "Yes."

Unbelievable! She'd weigh me, look at my pathology report to see what kind of cancer I had, and then look up the kind of chemo best suited for my type of cancer (based on what, someone else?). She would have me look at wigs and get me started with chemo the following week. No additional blood work, no holistic treatment or supplement suggestions, no nutritional advice, no asking me about my lifestyle, no asking me about my history, no DNA testing. She was going to just look in her book to see what chemo was standard for my kind of cancer and then push me, fast, into treatments that very next week?

Wow, no way was I comfortable with this. I mean, *seriously!* When I meet with my clients about their health goals, I spend a lot of time with them. I ask them a lot of questions about their life, their diet, and health history, and I take a lot of time getting to know them in order to serve them to the best of my ability. I spend way more time with my clients than the oncologist did with me, and I had a life-threatening disease. I was really blown away.

I really did stay respectful towards her during our meeting, but what I learned in just that one half-hour meeting was incredible. I learned that she did not know about any of the holistic alternative treatments that I asked her about. She told me that she could not offer any sort of holistic options because she would lose her medical license if she made any suggestions. She also told me that they are not allowed to learn about any other treatments not supported by the AMA (American Medical Association) or the FDA (Federal Drug Administration). If she ever got caught making any recommendations other than what the AMA allows, she could be fired and lose her medical license.

This was eye-opening. I also learned that an oncologist's income is based primarily on the kickbacks they receive when they prescribe chemo to their patients — amounts as high as $10K per patient! No wonder they are very motivated to prescribe chemo treatments. This was alarming to me, and made me even more suspicious and annoyed with this entire industry. Yes, it is an industry.

The Cancer Industry: What I Wanted to Know and What You Need to Know

After the meeting with the oncologist, I wondered what the deal was with the medical industry and why there wasn't anything close to a cure for cancer, even though there appears to be billions of dollars being poured into research. Why aren't more holistic and alternative treatments offered? I needed a dumbed-down explanation to understand why this was taking place. *The Flexner Report of 1910* explains it all.

The Flexner Report of 1910

Back in the early 1900s, there were many different options for medical care. There were holistic schools and medical schools. Both types of schools were well-promoted. Then the Rockefeller and Carnegie foundations decided they could make more money off a single unified approach to medicine. They created a medical monopoly to get rid of the competition. They patented all the chemical and medical educational systems. This was *The Flexner Report of 1910,* a book-length study of medical education written by "independent" sources under the aegis of the Rockefellers and the Carnegies.

The outcome of this "report" meant that any colleges and schools that were not pushing enough chemicals and drugs manufactured by Rockefeller and Carnegie were shut down. The AMA started shutting down all the larger homeopathic colleges. Carnegie and Rockefeller starting pouring in millions of dollars to the remaining medical schools, most of which were teaching drug-intensive medicine. This is why medical schools today are not teaching holistic practices. They are funded by pharmaceutical drug companies.

By 1923, the 22 homeopathic 'medical' schools that had flourished in the 1900s had dwindled to just two.

By 1925, over 10,000 herbalists were out of business.

By 1940, over 1,500 chiropractors would be prosecuted for practicing "quackery."

By 1950, all schools teaching homeopathy were closed.

In an article written by Dr. Darrel Wolfe, he says: "If a physician did not graduate from a 'Flexner-approved' medical school and receive an M.D. degree, then he or she could not find a job. This is why today M.D.'s are so heavily biased toward synthetic drug therapy and know little about nutrition, if anything. They don't even study what makes a healthy body; they study disease. Modern doctors are taught virtually nothing about nutrition, gentle daily cleansing, wellness, or disease prevention. Expecting a medical doctor to guide you on health issues is sort of like expecting your local butcher to perform surgery on you. It's simply not an area in which they have been trained.

"Since *The Flexner Report* was released, have we seen any progress? 100 years ago, if a medical doctor saw a case of cancer he would call on his colleagues because it was felt that they may never see this again, since cancer was so rare. Diabetes was practically unheard of, atherosclerosis (hardening of the arteries) was nonexistent, and the term "heart attack" hadn't even been coined yet."

This made sense to me. I've had many clients who were doctors and worked with me to learn about nutrition, and I was always curious as to why they were always more prone to prescribe medications and push vaccines. Now I understood. Most M.D.'s don't study what makes a body healthy, they study disease, because this is what they are taught in medical school. Learning this gave me confidence and helped me understand that cancer doctors were not going to be helpful in supporting my choice of using alternative treatments. They are biased. They are not truly treating disease. In actuality, they are partly promoting it. This is why I had to become my own health advocate and seek out natural alternative treatments and therapies. This, for me, was my only option for the outcome I wanted, which was to cure my cancer and not have it come back.

The other part of this is the cancer research side. Billions of dollars are poured into cancer research, but despite all the fake claims that they've made breakthroughs, cancer has continued to increase and there still is no cure through traditional treatments.

The reason why is because there is a lot of profit in keeping people sick. Cancer research is covering up much of the evidence, evidence like research studies proving that the primary cause of cancer is toxins. Those who produce toxins and sell toxic products are not being exposed.

Researcher and health advocate Tony Isaacs writes, "In fact the BCAM, one of the biggest movements to support breast cancer, was created by the Imperial Chemical Company, now bought out by AstraZeneca, which are the largest known producers of carcinogens in the US. So in other words, to ensure the spotlight is kept off toxins, cancer-causing companies have placed representatives in key positions in both government agencies and non-profit organizations. These include the National Cancer Institute, the American Cancer Society (ACS), and the Breast Cancer Awareness Movement."

Then there is greed.

How Greed Drives the Cancer Industry

The industry of cancer has grown to be a financial monster that includes all of the inside workers: the doctors, nurses, technicians, labs, hospitals, and chemotherapy drug makers. Also included are the huge salaries given as well as the perks and expenses in government agencies and non-profits. The doomed reality is that all of these financial profits, salaries, and perks will continue to increase, and the medical industry that can't cure cancer generates revenues in excess of $95.5 billion per year.

You think the infamous "Pink Ribbon" organization uses their profits for holistic research? Far from it. Their profits go largely to their enormous executive salaries and to "education" and "awareness" campaigns that lead to the push for more mammograms. An article written by *The Truth About Cancer* organization states, "How can an organization that claims to be focused on preventing and curing breast cancer partner with companies that sell highly processed fast food, junk food, artificial food, hormone-filled dairy products, and sugar/chemical-laden food and beverages that have had a strong correlation with contributing to cancer?" I personally think that the Environmental Working Group (EWG) is a far better charitable organization to support if you are interested in learning about ways to support your cancer fight.

If you are a little fired up right now, you should be. Now you know that the medical cancer industry doesn't have your best interest at heart. The reason why this pertains to you and why you need to understand it, is because alternative treatments are being hidden from you. Many holistic clinics have been shut down and interrogated by the FDA (read up about the Hoxsey Clinics and how they were shut down by the FDA, AMA, and NCI because they were taking a different approach in healing cancer naturally and with great success). These government entities did not like clinic founder Harry Hoxsey because his protocol did not fit into the "narrative of the medical establishment," and they made sure the clinics were shut down. I strongly recommend you read about this. It will make you sick when you learn what they did to this poor man, who was doing nothing but curing people of cancer. So, what did Harry do? He moved all his clinics to Mexico. This is what he had to do.

Understanding the history of why alternative medicine isn't promoted or tolerated here in the US is important for you to understand because there *is* a cure for cancer using holistic methods, total lifestyle changes, and nutrition. These treatments are not toxic or poisonous. But the big problem is that they are not covered under our medical insurance, which is a huge bummer and the reason why so many opt for the standard treatments today. You can go and get chemo and radiation and all the medicines that cost hundreds of thousands of dollars, but to work with an alternative doctor for your cancer treatment? It's not going to be covered by insurance. So more than likely, it's not going to happen. You can see why so many resort to oncologists and current allopathic treatments for their care, because those are covered by medical insurance.

Many people struggle with how to afford working with a holistic M.D. This is a huge problem in our medical system today. The current medical system is broken. Why would insurance pay thousands of dollars for chemo but not a penny for any holistic treatment, holistic device, or supplements? If we are sick and want to use alternative methods, our medical system will say, nope, sorry, you have to use our methods of treatment if you want it covered. Otherwise, you're on your own. You see the problem? Many people are forced financially to make a decision they don't want. I was fortunate to have amazing parents who helped fund my alternative treatment, and I was lucky to find and benefit from working with a holistic M.D. If you can't afford one, it's imperative that you educate yourself and seek out support.

About five months into my journey of healing myself of cancer, I decided to find a holistic doctor, one who could advise me how to step up my healing protocols and administer holistic treatments not offered by standard medicine. I realized that I would not only learn more, but it would give me some additional peace of mind. This is when I reached out to Dr. Conners, founder of Conners Clinic in Minnesota. This man is brilliant, and was the one who got me started on the Rife Machine (I talk about this treatment later on page 104). It was important for me to do whatever I could, from all angles, to try protocols and treatments that were going to support my immune system, and not destroy it. Dr. Conners did some very targeting DNA testing that was specialized and customized for me.

The additional peace of mind I gained by knowing he was going to oversee my entire treatment was comforting. In addition, he was able to teach me about my own DNA profile, which was crucial in determining how to best support my own genes to fight my cancer. He was thorough, confident, intelligent, and absolutely the most well-educated doctor I had ever met. It was important that I trust everyone that I was going to work with moving forward, because the previous doctors I'd had made mistakes and weren't up to speed on the latest research. Dr. Conners had my trust, and still does to this day. In addition, he is an amazing human being. I loved learning from him. He was truly a Godsend.

The other main research point for you to take time to really understand is: What is cancer? I've been lied to; you've been lied to. I was assuming and hearing that cancer was a death sentence. So I had to step back and commit to really understanding what cancer was so that I could make a decision that was not based on fear and pressure. I had to *slow down* and get past the initial shock of the news. I had to learn as much as I could about how my body worked so I could start to implement the right treatments. I think, if you do this, you will find a huge sense of power and relief like I did. I learned that cancer does not have to be a death sentence if you do the right things to heal your body.

What is cancer? Cancer is a disease. It is caused by an uncontrolled division of abnormal cells in a part of the body. There are many different things that cause these cells to divide and become unhealthy, and we will get into this later in the upcoming chapters. What you need to understand is that we all have cancer cells present in our bodies, however, they are typically recognized by our immune systems and destroyed before they cause any problems. It is when the cancer cells go unrecognized by the immune system that they begin to multiply. So we must figure out what steps we can take to eliminate cancer-causing agents and change our lifestyles. We also need to build up our immune systems to be able to recognize cancer cells and fight them. Chemo and radiation destroy our immune systems, and they also kill our good cells that fight for us. You really don't want to destroy what your body is designed to do, do you?

Once I understood that cancer was simply a disease and not a death sentence, I had hope. You see, I have helped hundreds of clients reverse, control, and eradicate disease. I'd just never thought about cancer like this before. Thinking of cancer as "just a disease" was eye-opening for me. I realized, "I can reverse my disease. I have done this before with myself and my clients, now I just have to learn how to do it with cancer." So I did. And now I'm going to teach you.

Another thing I learned that blew me away is that a tumor, in and of itself, is not dangerous, but rather the cells that can break off from it. The tumor itself rarely kills people unless it grows big enough to block or obstruct some major airway or organ. It's the metastatic process that is dangerous, in which circulating tumor cells (CTCs) that have detached from the primary tumor get into the bloodstream and create secondary tumors. This is metastasis, and, fascinatingly, this is what your immune system is designed to attack and *kill*. This is why oncologists whose primary concern is to remove or shrink a tumor are following the wrong approach. It's imperative to go after the cancer stem cells. This is why chemo and radiation make your cancer worse, because 1) they don't kill the cancer stem cells, 2) if you don't address the cancer stem cells, the cancer will come back, and 3) they can cause secondary cancers.

Tumors cells don't metastasize. The cancer stem cells metastasize. The cancer stem cells are actually *resistant* to chemo and radiation; it makes no sense to use these modalities to try and eradicate them. In fact, the latest research from Harvard Medical School and UCLA shows that chemo actually stimulates cancer stem cells, which then become the germ cells from which new tumors arise. So, ask your oncologist when you see him/her, "What are we going to do to kill the CTCs?" Sadly, they will not know what to say. They are not up to speed on the latest research. They are still focused on shrinking tumors, not killing CTCs.

Everyone who has cancer has CTCs, and they are only kept dormant by a healthy immune system. Chemo and radiation wreck our immune systems and increase the risk of more cancer. Why aren't oncologists or mainstream media telling us this? Think about it. The cancer industry (i.e., standard oncology) makes their moolah by selling cancer therapies that may kill cancer cells, but not CTCs. A recent University of Michigan study reveals that for many cancer patients who use chemotherapy, there is an increase in CTCs following the treatment, which is why the cancer comes back with a vengeance and in a short period of time. If oncology would start addressing CTCs, then it would greatly impact their profits from standard cancer treatments.

If you take away anything from this book, please, please understand this. Your immune systems is what kills CTCs, *not* chemo and radiation. Do you get this? I mean, really get this? Seriously, this is what you must understand and believe if you truly want to heal your body. Can you see that if you know how to build your cancer-fighting immune system, you will have less likelihood and fear of your cancer coming back? You will never, ever hear this from your oncologist. Makes you truly think, doesn't it?

Cancer Is a Reversible Disease

This is how you should think of your cancer: as a disease, a disease you can reverse. Of course, I can't make claims, nor do I want to. All I am saying is that this is what worked for me, this is how I cured my cancer. It was hard. I am not going to lie. I had to change my entire way of thinking, eating, managing stress, the products I used, who I associated with, and much more. It was not an easy process, but, pick your "hard." Was what I did harder than chemo? Let's see. With chemo, I would have been sick all of the time; I would have ruined my immune system; I would have lost my hair; damaged the good cells in my body; had side effects that lasted far beyond the chemo treatments; and lived in fear that the chemo might kill me. So, which is harder? I'll take the holistic hard any day.

It was the best decision for me, for sure. Not only did I reverse my disease, but I became an all-around healthier person, feeling the best I have ever felt my entire life, and I learned so much along the way. The entire experience really did change me for the better. I can say this now, but looking back to the first two months of the treatments and waiting to see if everything I was doing was working, was very emotionally challenging and difficult. But again: harder than chemo/radiation? I don't think so! I am just so very glad that I am here today writing to you about how I healed my cancer and how I was able to have a really good quality of life while treating myself holistically, versus writing to you about how to get through agonizing treatments and side effects. Ugh. I just want to cry when I hear about people who decide to go that route.

When I really sit back and reflect on the whole journey, from the day I noticed the lump in my neck until the day I got the call that I no longer had any cancer, it was 13 months. Thirteen months is a long time when you are battling for your health, fighting the medical mainstream, wrestling with creative money management, and contending with the mind games that go on every single day. But, honestly? I truly believe I was picked to go through this so I could help others. I mean, who was better equipped to be put to this test? Me? I think so. I went through it, and because I did, I understand fully what it's like. I can now empathize, educate, help, coach, and mentor so much more compassionately and effectively. For that, I am grateful, and I want to give back to you in any way that I can to make this process a relatively uncomplicated one for you.

Little did you know that you are already doing STEP 1 of the REFUSED Solution, by reading this book. Congratulations! You are on your way to making an important decision on your journey to health. Most people who work with me directly, whether to survive cancer, overcome disease, or to recover from other debilitating symptoms, have found such huge relief in not having to go through all the time, energy, and challenges of researching and coming up with a plan on their own. I help make it easier for them because I've done most of the research already. So, great job on taking one step closer to getting your power back and healing your cancer.

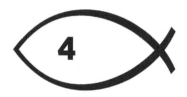

4

E — ENVIRONMENTAL TOXINS

"You cannot kill cancer with chemotherapy, radiation, and surgery alone.

You must do other immune stimulating therapies and search for the cause."

– Dr. Kevin Conners

t was a Friday afternoon a few weeks after my birthday, and I decided to use some of my birthday money to go get my hair done. I wanted to get all dolled up and get the real overhaul. I was going to get highlights, get my hair extensions tightened (don't judge — ha), and get a haircut. But this visit was surreal. I had a pit in my stomach the entire day before and even during the appointment itself.

You see, this was about two months before my surgery to remove the lymph node. Up until this point, I really wasn't thinking it was cancer. But deep down I kept worrying, "What if it is cancer?" This also was before I went into full research mode. I still did not even know what my options would be if I "did" have cancer, so I wasn't well-researched. I think I was still not wanting to face the what-ifs. This hair appointment, however, put those thoughts right in my face: "If I have cancer, then this will be my last hair appointment." The only thing I could do that entire hair appointment was think to myself, "I might not have hair. I might lose all of my hair that has taken me years to grow out. I wonder if they have wigs that would look similar to my style?" The thought of wearing a wig was horrifying. The thought of being bald was mortifying.

I kept thinking about the actress Shannon Doherty, from *Beverly Hills 90210,* who had been recently diagnosed with cancer, was doing chemo, and was having quite the battle. She explained in an article she wrote that after only her second treatment, her hair got really matted, and when she tried to brush it, huge clumps of hair landed in her hands. She cried, "My hair, my hair, my hair!" I started tearing up sitting in the styling chair, hoping that Aimee wouldn't notice and ask me what was wrong. Thinking about this, and wondering, "Will this be me? Will this be my last hair appointment? Will my hair ever grow back the same color, texture?" You see, the reason Shannon came to mind was because when she was diagnosed, it had hit me hard. I used to watch her on TV. She was about my age, and very healthy looking, fit, and beautiful, but the treatments, for a time, were really taking a toll on her appearance. I didn't want that to happen to me. It scared me so much!

I don't know about you, but when I'm scared, I seek out knowledge. When I first learned about the deadliness of CTCs and their resistance to chemo, I knew my best chance at healing was to boost my immune system. I also knew that I needed to understand the factors that contribute to the formation of cancer cells so I could start to change my lifestyle. I didn't realize how influential environmental toxins were in the formation of cancer — way more than I imagined. This was eye opening. Here are some of these key environmental hazards.

GMOs

GMOs are Genetically Modified Organisms. They are everywhere. Want holes in your stomach, want leaky gut, want to encourage the growth of cancer cells? Then put GMOs in your body. A GMO is the result of a laboratory process in which genes from the DNA of one species are extracted and artificially forced into the genes of an unrelated plant or animal. The foreign genes may come from bacteria, viruses, insects, animals, or even humans. There are two kinds of GMOs. The first type is a pesticide producer: they take a gene from bacteria in the soil and it's injected into a plant so that when a bug tries to eat it, a toxin is released, creating a hole in their gut and causing them to die. Problem is, when we eat foods that have this toxin in it, it is doing the same thing to us: creating holes in our guts. Our guts are a huge part of our immune system. And remember, our immune system is what kills cancer.

The second type of GMO is an herbicide resistor: this is most familiar to you as a product called Roundup, designed to make plants immune to the weed killer produced by the same company. Thanks to Roundup Resistance, when weed killers are sprayed on crops, they don't kill the plant. Instead, the herbicides are soaked up inside of the plants. There are several scientific studies that prove Roundup causes tumors as well as liver, kidney, and gastrointestinal damage.

The AAEM (American Academy of Environmental Medicine) has studies that indicate serious health risks from GMOs, and yet we are surrounded by these products. They are in pretty much anything in a package, all fast food, and anything that is non-organic. Top GMO products and ingredients include corn, soy (lecithin), aspartame, high fructose corn Syrup, and canola oil, to name just a few. I wrote a blog post about it, and you can find the link in the back of this book.

The list of diseases and dysfunctions in the body due to ingesting GMOs is very long. I encourage you to do your own research on this; what you will learn will be very eye-opening. Jeffrey Smith is a GMO expert and the head of the Institute of Responsible Technology. If you want to learn about this in detail, I recommend watching his film called *Genetic Roulette*.

Environmental Toxins

Did you know that environmental toxins are all around us? There are environmental pollutants everywhere we turn. Many of them are carcinogenic (carcinogen: a physical, chemical, or biological agent that causes cancerous growth in the body). They are in our soil (see GMOs, above), our water, and our food supply.

One of the most harmful substances in our food supply is an excitotoxin called MSG. This toxin actually excites brain cells to death. Dr. Blaylock is an author, retired neurosurgeon, and researcher. He explains how MSG (monosodium glutamate) destroys brain cells. But his research and studies also show that every cell in the body has glutamate receptors, not just the brain. What that means is when you ingest glutamate, all the cells in your body are being exposed. Your blood levels rises very rapidly and stay very high for a prolonged period of time. When this happens, the glutamate receptors trigger and stimulate the growth and invasion of cancers of every kind. What Dr. Blaylock found is that if you have high glutamate levels around a tumor, the tumor becomes highly invasive and grows twice as fast as a tumor that has low glutamate levels. So glutamate acts as a fertilizer and stimulant for cancer. There are some natural glutamate blockers that you should be aware of. They are resveratrol, curcumin, quercetin, ellagic acid, and flavonoids (compounds found in plants).

Some other environmental toxins that are listed as carcinogenic and harmful are surprisingly listed on the National Cancer Institute's website. They are:

- ✓ Substances in the environment and workplace, such as air pollutants, water pollutants, and chemicals. (For example, the Diesel Exhaust in Miners Study found that heavy exposure to diesel exhaust is associated with an increased risk of lung cancer.)

- ✓ Infectious agents, such as viruses and bacteria. (The Study to Understand Cervical Cancer Early Endpoints and Determinants, for example, aims to distinguish which women with human papillomavirus infections are at highest risk of cervical cancer.)

- ✓ Radiation, including ionizing radiation and non-ionizing radiation. (DCEG investigators are involved in several studies of cancer incidence among children undergoing CT scans.)

- ✓ Pharmaceutical agents and exogenous and endogenous hormones. (Researchers involved in the DES Follow-Up Study, for example, are following diethylstilbestrol-exposed and unexposed mothers and their daughters, sons, and granddaughters for adverse health effects, including cancer.)

✓ Behavioral and lifestyle factors, such as diet and nutrition, tobacco use, alcohol use, energy balance, physical activity, and obesity. (DCCPS' <u>Transdisciplinary Research on Energetics and Cancer</u> <u>Exit Disclaimer</u> initiative funds research in this area.)

✓ Immune system status and inflammation. (DCEG researchers are studying how chronic inflammation from Helicobacter pylori infection is related to gastric cancer risk.)

If you were to break down everything from the points above, it would include items like fungi in our food, arsenic, asbestos, clothing dyes, PVC plastic, second-hand smoke, formaldehyde, aluminum (found in deodorants), oxybenzone (a chemical added to sunscreens), chemicals used in Teflon cookware, chemicals used in hand soaps, parabens (used in shampoos and perfumes), and toxic agents that are used in carpeting and rugs. The list is so long, it is overwhelming. It makes you think that nothing is safe anymore. The things we put *in, on,* and *around* us are full of toxic agents known to have cancer-causing properties.

BPA/Plastics

The next time you grab a bottled water, think twice. BPA, also known as Bisphenol A, is a powerful xenoestrogen found in most plastic bottles, containers, and canned products. This is a proven hormone disrupter and has been strongly linked to causing cancer, especially breast cancer. The reason is because BPA is known to leach into the water when exposed to heat (sunlight, microwave, etc.), which in return creates a bad estrogen. (A "bad" estrogen is also known as a xenoestrogen. This basically is a fancy name for a man-made estrogen made from our external environment, usually from dangerous chemical substances. Other names for xenoestrogens would be "estrogen mimickers" and "endocrine disrupters.") High levels of the "bad" estrogen in the body have been shown to cause ovarian, prostate, and breast cancers.

Polyethylene Terephthalate (PET)

PET bottles are BPA-free, but they pose other potential health risks. According to studies by North Dakota State University, PET bottles contain contaminants of fecal matter, saliva, and food residues in the plastic, so they are hazardous to your health when re-used. This is primarily because the soft plastic is nearly impossible to clean, setting the stage for the significant presence of contaminants after multiple usage.

Phthalates

Phthalates are another chemical compound used to make plastic flexible, particularly PVC (polyvinyl chloride). These also leach into the water contained in their bottles or water supplied by PVC pipes. The problems they cause in humans include liver cancer, testicular atrophy, and sterility in males. The jury is still out on this one, but there have been many studies strongly suggesting a relationship between these compounds and cancer.

Drinking Water and Fluoride

Tap water contains bleach, fluoride, chlorine, and toxic metals like lead and copper. Our municipalities put chlorine in our drinking water to kill harmful bacteria. They put a chemical in our water to neutralize our drinking water so it won't rust the water pipes, and then it is absorbed by our bodies. Then they put fluoride in our water because they "think" that it is good for our teeth. Fluoride is actually one of the most toxic agents we can consume. Daniel Nuzum, NMD, DO, DN, is both a certified doctor of natural medicine as well as a medical acupuncturist and says that "fluoride toxicity causes the bones to dissolve. It actually causes the teeth to dissolve. Fluoride rots our bones and they become soft and brittle. Fluoride has been linked to bone cancer (osteocarcoma)." Scientific studies have proven that fluoride causes dental fluorosis, brain damage, birth defects, and osteoporosis. Have you ever read the warning label on a tube of toothpaste? It will disturb you. The following warning is required an all fluoridated toothpaste by the FDA since April of 1997 due to the large number of calls to the Poison Control Centers for children who became acutely ill from ingested sodium fluoride: "WARNING: Keep out of reach of children under 6 years of age. In case of accidental overdose, seek professional assistance or contact a poison control center immediately."

Fluoride is a poison and mutagen (a chemical agent causing mutations). Fluoride chemicals inflict the type of genetic damage that later on down the road can trigger the formation of cancer. I bet you won't ever drink tap water again.

Chlorine

Chlorine is poisonous. It is put in our water to kill potentially harmful microorganisms and water-borne diseases. It is being put in our water supply and, most commonly, swimming pools and hot tubs. Chlorine is definitely as hazardous as fluoride. It would seem to me, if it is supposed to kill harmful microorganisms, wouldn't this be a pesticide? To me this is common sense, but then why are we being told it is safe? Again, more studies, like the Breast Cancer Research Study (Hartford, CT), find 50-60% higher levels of chlorination in the breast tissue of women with breast cancer than women without breast cancer. Also, the U.S. Council of Environmental Quality has this to say: "Cancer risk among people drinking chlorinated water is 93% higher than among those whose water does not contain chlorine."

Body Care Products

Remember, your skin is your largest organ, so whatever you put on it is going to be absorbed into your bloodstream and circulate throughout your entire body — lotions, makeup, oils, soaps, perfumes, etc. Some of the most toxic ingredients on the market are used in skin care.

Vaccines

I understand this is a very controversial topic. My entire purpose of writing this book is to share with you what I did and what I researched in order to better understand what might have been a contributor to my cancer. I really wanted to know. Although I will never know the exact combination of things that caused it, I can tell you this: There were quite a few things that I learned I needed to change in my lifestyle that were causing suppression of my immune system and were potential contributors in the developing of my cancer.

Whatever your position is on vaccines, I recommend researching them from both perspectives and then coming to your own conclusions. Here is what I know. The media and the CDC (Centers for Disease Control) are not sharing this information with you. Vaccine manufacturers do not want you to know the truth, because the truth would affect their profits. Here are the facts. Ingredients in vaccines include aluminum, formaldehyde, MSG, mercury, hydrocortisone, chicken cells/ DNA, eggs and egg residue from the manufacturing process, detergents, triton x-100, gelatin, MDCK cells/dog DNA from kidneys, chicken stealth viruses — *yuck!* If you go to the www.fda.gov website, you can download an actual product package inserts for any of the vaccines. Also, if you go to the Center for Disease Controls website (www.cdc.gov/vaccines) you can get an itemized list of all the ingredients that are in every vaccine. Quite honestly, after you go and look at what is in a vaccine and read up on the dangers and side effects of the toxic ingredients, I will be very surprised if you will ever want to get another vaccine. Here is a visual that lists the many ingredients that are in a majority of vaccines.

Vaccine Ingredients

Multiple vaccines are frequently given in just one visit.
Dosage is not modified for age, weight, or health of individual.

Ingredients	Amount Per Shot
Yeast Protein (Fungus)	35,000 mcg
Aluminum (Neurotoxin)	5,700 mcg
Formaldehyde (Carcinogen, Embalming Agent)	801.6 mcg
Urea (Waste From Human Urine)	5,000 mcg
Gelatin (Ground Up Animal Carcasses)	23,250 mcg
Human Albumin (Human Blood)	500 mcg
2-Phenoxyethanol (Antifreeze)	17,500 mcg
Mono-Sodium L-Glutamate (MSG: Exotoxin Causing Obesity)	760 mcg
Polysorbate-80 (Carcinogen)	560 mcg
Potassium Phosphate (Liquid Fertilizer Agent)	188 mcg
Benzethonium Chloride (Toxic Agent)	**
Thimerosol (Mercury)	**
Antibiotics	**
2-Phenolxyethanol (Antibacterial Agent/Insect Repellent)	**
Glutaraldehyde (Disinfectant)	**

Ingredients and mcg amounts vary by vaccine
** Unknown and/or trace amounts**

Precautions: Some of the side effects of the ingredients listed above are; Chest pains and tightness, arrhythmias, inflammation, kidney damage, autism, encephalitis, eczema, fever, paralysis, seizures, asthma, diarrhea, cough, chills, permanent brain damage and death. (to name a few)

For ingredients list visit:
www.cdc.gov/vaccines/pubs/pinkbook/downloads/
appendices/B/excipient-table-2.pdf

For side effects of vaccines, visit:
www.cdc.gov/vaccines/vac-gen/side-effects.htm

For even more in depth info, visit:
vaxtruth.org/2011/08/vaccine-ingredients/

To read up on how vaccines affect your immune system, visit:
www.vaccineinjury.com

Mercury causes cancer. No ifs, ands, or buts about it. I also learned from Dr. Conners that a vaccine I had years ago, back when I was too young to make these decisions myself, was a major contributor to the development of my specific cancer. I had a targeted DNA test done that showed I was not able to detox this particular vaccine. Not good! It affected my cells and my detoxing pathways. I am not going to go into details about this because it is extremely difficult to even explain, and quite honestly, it is way over my head, but when the DNA test showed this and Dr. Conners explained it to me, it made me mad and confirmed my decision to never get another vaccine. You will ultimately have to make your own educated decision and do your own research. Every cancer patient should have their DNA tested by someone who understands how DNA testing works, and who understands how your body is functioning. This process is key in learning how to heal your cancer and how to proceed with lifelong nutrition and supplemental adjustments for best health.

"As far as real science is concerned, there is no evidence that you should vaccinate yourself or your children, ever, for any reason. I am well

aware that vaccines are considered 'sacred' to most physicians. As a matter of fact, questioning them is tantamount to blasphemy. I can assure you that I would not challenge the efficacy and safety of something as 'holy' as vaccines unless I were certain, beyond a shadow of a doubt, that I am accurate when I state that vaccines are not safe (unless you change the definition of 'safe' to include death, numerous diseases, and brain damage). The greatest lie ever told is that vaccines are safe and effective."

– Dr. Len Horowitz

But don't take Dr. Horowitz's word for it! Check out the statistics for yourself. From 1990 to 2008, the US Government recorded 238,755 vaccine-related injuries and deaths, according to the Vaccine Adverse Event Reporting System (VAERS) database. Since the FDA estimates that 90% of vaccine reactions go unrecorded, we can extrapolate that during the past 18 years, there have actually been almost 2.4 million vaccine related injuries and deaths, as quoted in the illuminating documentary *Vaxxed: From Cover-Up to Catastrophe.*

Bottom line, formaldehyde has been related to head and neck cancers, myeloid leukemia, and lymphomas. Breast cancer, neuroblastoma, and tumors in the lung and cervix are all also associated with the stray viruses that are in vaccines.

*****

One of every three women and one of two men will be diagnosed with cancer. The odds of getting cancer are higher than ever before, and I am convinced that what is around is, what we put in us, and what we put on us, are the reasons why as a society we are getting sicker and sicker.

Am I losing you? I understand this seems very overwhelming, and when I first started out, I didn't know any of this stuff, either. I also felt extremely agitated that our government is really not telling us everything we need to know in order to stay healthy and happy. It is our responsibility to be our own health advocates. I know it seems backwards, but that is just the world we are living in now. I am sure you are feeling like "everything seems to give us cancer and disease, so what's the point?" I understand; it sure seems that way. But I think if you truly want to improve your health or heal cancer or any other disease (which I believe you do want to do, or you wouldn't be reading this book), then I would just take all this information and use it as a way to take some action.

At first, small steps: Pick one or two things you can start to do immediately. You know your situation and your surroundings better than anyone, so if something jumped out at you, then take that as a sign to start there. You do not have to do everything all at once. Just take this information and take the time to do your own research for you and your family and decide if this is where you'd like to start. You don't have to feel bad, you didn't know. Neither did I. We have been lied to. So, it's time for a restart: a fresh start in deciding which lifestyle changes you will start to implement in your healing plan, one day — and one thing — at a time. Here are some great places to start.

Action Steps

1) **Stop eating fast food.** Every single fast food chain uses GMOs in their foods. A blog article by Deborah Oke breaks down all of the ingredients in a McDonald's Big

Mac, listing 91 ingredients that are toxic and harmful to your health. That's just in *one* hamburger, and doesn't even include the pop and fries and condiments that you eat along with it!

2) **Stop using plastic bottles, and especially bottled water.** Even when it's supposedly been "filtered" (and how would you really know?), water in plastic bottles is full of BPA and phthalates known to disrupt your endocrine systems. You also want to avoid using anything plastic when microwaving or exposing to heat. For example, don't leave plastic bottles out in the hot sun. Use glass jars for your liquids and glass containers to store and heat your food. A note about canned food: can liners also contain BPA, so if a specific canned food is acidic in nature, like tomato products, the BPA has been proven to leak out — even with organic foods.

3) **Get a home water filtration system.** Do your research. Do not drink tap water. I own a Kangen Water System, which I absolutely love, but there are definitely cheaper systems out there. You can also check out reverse osmosis systems and water purifiers. These systems will remove contaminants like bacteria and parasites, as well as fluoride, chlorine, arsenic, lead, mercury, and pharmaceutical drugs that leak into the water supply.

4) **Consider a shower and bath filtration system**. Most of us have to pick our battles and do our best to make the changes that are best suited for our budgets. I own an Aquasana Deluxe Shower Water Filter System for my shower and a separate filter for my bathtub. They work great, and I feel good knowing that I don't have all those harmful chemicals soaking into my skin.

5) **Use pool and hot tub filtration.** If you have a pool or hot tub, consider using a silver-copper ion generator or looking into organic solutions. There are a bunch of good ones out there just a Google search away.

6) **Switch to an organic toothpaste**. You do not want to be brushing with fluoride.

7) **Use organic body lotions and personal care products.** We must omit our toxic overload, and these products are being absorbed into our systems and causing a lot of endocrine disruption as well as cancer. Being exposed to these toxins and chemicals just makes it harder for our immune systems to fight the cancer. Do your best to take steps in cleaning up your environment to promote health and healing.

If you're overwhelmed by how to find the right foods and products, check out www.ewg.org. I visit there regularly to check on many products and foods. They have a huge list of products and their ingredients. This is a great resource for you to search for your particular item, learn what is in it, and how toxic it is.

Because everyone is different and has different environmental exposures, I make it a priority to help each of my clients discern what environmental toxins are most important for them to avoid. My client Kris, for example, started having problems with bloating and stomach pain. She was eating a healthy diet, or so she thought, so when she described her symptoms to me, I immediately put on my detective hat and took a deep look at where she was spending time, what she was ingesting, and whether she'd recently made any changes in her topical products, etc.

After a few weeks of trying different things, I asked her what she was using for protein drinks and what she was putting in them. When she told me she was using a specific brand of almond milk, I immediately thought, "DING DING DING!" The particular brand of almond milk she was buying was not an organic brand, and it had an ingredient in there that was heavily processed and considered toxic. She was having a strong reaction to this one ingredient. We pulled her off of that brand right away, and within a week, she was feeling better.

So many times we are putting toxins into our body and we don't even realize they are causing inflammatory responses and symptoms that can potentially, over time, develop into chronic illnesses. This is why it's important to always listen to your body and find someone who is experienced in nutrition to help you.

I understand all of this information can feel overwhelming, but it is important that you start somewhere, because we are surrounded by toxins literally at every turn. When we come up with an Environmental Toxin Elimination plan, we can move forward and make positive changes for you and your situation.

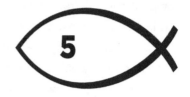

F — FOOD

Genesis 1:29 — Then God said, "I give you every seed-bearing plant on the face of the whole earth and every tree that has fruit with seed in it. They will be yours for food."

"Let food be thy medicine and medicine be thy food."

– Hippocrates

Thanksgiving is one of my favorite holidays. Especially that Thanksgiving meal: turkey, mashed potatoes, stuffing, yams, corn, and, for dessert, pumpkin pie. It was the holiday meal of the year I enjoyed the most. But the year I had cancer, my Thanksgiving meal was anything but enjoyable. I recall my mom asking me the week before, "Teri, is there anything I can make for you that you can eat?" I told her it would be easier if I made my own food and brought it with me. And it was.

But it also made me feel left out and frustrated that I couldn't enjoy the wonderful food on the table. I mean, the smell of the turkey was amazing. The candied yams with melted marshmallow topping were my absolute favorite. The green beans with mushrooms, cheese, and onion rings — ugh, so good. I was so tempted to just to say, "Screw it, I'm gonna splurge today." But I knew that if I did that, I would be disappointed in myself and know that it would not be helping with my healing process. Extreme? Well, yes — and no. I had cancer, and I would not give in. And you know what that discipline did for me? Healed my cancer in nine months. No regrets! But this Thanksgiving? Oh, yes, I will be making up for last year!

Memorial Day, birthday parties, graduations, the Fourth of July, Christmas, and yes, my favorite holiday, Thanksgiving, were all events I attended where I brought my own food, bringing my own cooler with me or eating before I went. Yep, I did it. I was serious. I had cancer; this was not something to take lightly. I made a decision to go holistic. I had to radically change my nutrition, first and foremost.

I recall numerous times when I would be at appointments, carrying my medicinal mushrooms or matcha green tea to sip on throughout the day. There was never a time when someone didn't make a comment about my drink. It did look like mud in a jar, and they would make sure to remind me of that. My comment back, *every time*, was, "Well, I will choose this over chemo any day. It's healing my body." Then they'd shut up.

Every time I was tempted to go off my anti-cancer plan, I just immediately thought of the other option, which was *not* healing my cancer. I would always be visualizing my body healing itself.

Was it easy? No. Did I cheat? Honestly, *no!* Was it worth it? *100% yes!* Guys, in nine months, I had a clean PET scan. What I put in my body was key to my healing.

Everything I read and researched; everyone I talked to that had healed their cancers; everything I heard from Dr. Conners, told me that nutrition was the first thing I needed to change. I did know this already, because as a functional diagnostic nutritionist I had seen the power of nutrition, supplements, and lifestyle change in many of my clients. But it was still powerful validation and reinforcement. I knew that the food I put in my body was my medicine, and I ended up feeling incredibly great during the process. It was really amazing.

If you want to really get into the chemical nature of food and how it works, I strongly suggest reading Patrick Quillin's *Beating Cancer with Nutrition*. His book gives you detailed, scientific insight on how nutrition can cure your cancer. But I also want to simplify it for you. I'm going to help you understand that what you eat, how you eat, and where you eat will determine whether or not you create an environment for your body to heal. I think this is, by far, the number one area of importance for anyone diagnosed with cancer to start addressing immediately. Food does not require a prescription and is very easy to get. Food is our medicine.

Our culture has gotten so used to eating for pleasure versus eating to survive and for health. People these days are obsessed with food and gluttony. I understand, we have taste buds for a reason, and sadly, unhealthy, genetically modified, processed foods are all very tasty and addictive, not to mention inexpensive and convenient. No wonder why we have the highest rates of obesity and sickness than ever before.

We now understand that GMOs are highly responsible for cancer growth and immune system suppression, so why are we putting them in our bodies? Because they taste good! But when we eat, we are either promoting health or promoting disease. All fast food, processed food and non-organic food causes an inflammatory response in our bodies, which is always one of the causes of cancer. Honestly, no one, cancer patients or not, should be eating any of this, because it is causing damage to us whether we know it or not. Depending on your own unique DNA, you might get sick sooner or later, but it will catch up with you. If you have cancer, it is imperative that you stop eating fast foods, GMOs, and sugar, immediately. Speaking of sugar....

Sugar

Sugar is a cancer feeder, and it is your enemy. Sugar is the absolute worst thing you can consume when you have cancer. Sugar is cancer's favorite food. Refined white sugar, brown sugar, and high fructose corn syrup are in pretty much every fast food item and most, if not all, packaged foods. Excess intake of any processed sugars results in compromised immune function (decreasing the white blood cells' ability to destroy bacteria), and, on a cellular level, causes cancer cells to grow. Stay away from sugar: any processed and packaged foods, cookies, cakes, candy bars, boxed juices, soda pop, syrups, jams, pastries, tabletop sugars, creamers, dairy products, refined flour — you get the idea. I'm sure you are wondering about the so called "healthy sugars," like honey, agave, coconut sugar, and fruits. Although you can get these unprocessed and they are very much healthier for you, sugar is still sugar, and sugar makes cancer cell stronger and bigger. As long as you have cancer, fruit consumption should be kept to a minimum, and, with some specific cancers and situations, avoided altogether. Again, to clarify, the nutritional value of fruit is beneficial, but too much fruit could be a cause for increased insulin production, which in some cases will not be ideal for a cancer patient. But the most important distinction will be eliminating the processed sugar. You will have to make your own decision on how much fruit you consume. I was very conservative with fruit, but did put a few berries in my green smoothies.

Animals Products: Meat

What about meat and dairy? No meat or dairy, of any kind, for now. Why? Meat and dairy promote cancer by elevating a growth hormone called IGF-1 (Insulin-like Growth Factor). IGF-1 is produced in your liver when you eat meat and dairy, and IGF-1 is directly linked to cancer growth. I was a huge protein eater. I loved protein shakes, chicken, eggs, and fish. I had to eat a lot of protein to accommodate my exercise load, so eliminating this was challenging for me. But it made sense. If you are trying to fight cancer, then you have to keep your IGF-1 levels down.

Still not sure? Let's talk about meat and how it pertains to cancer growth and healing. First of all, did you know that the FDA estimates that 24.6 million pounds of antibiotics are used, per year for "non-therapeutic purposes" — that is, to make animals grow to market weight faster and to prevent disease prevalent in the close quarters of confinement agriculture? Yes, over 80% of antibiotics sold are used on the animals we consume, exposing us to high levels of those antibiotics every time we eat meat. (Let me clarify that I am not referring to organic meat. USDA organic meats are not treated with any hormones and/or antibiotics. But even so, if you have cancer, for now, due to the increase in IGF-1, when you eat meat, you should not be eating any meat for a few weeks on your nutrition protocol).

Factory farms raising chickens, cows, pigs, and fish are motivated to produce high quantity, and quickly. These animals are crammed by the thousands into filthy sheds, cages, and crates where they cannot move around or comfortably breathe. They are being treated in an inhumane way. They are being injected with growth hormone to make them grow faster, and being genetically manipulated to produce more milk or eggs than they normally would. Most chickens grow so unnaturally big that they can't even stand, and they suffer tremendously. The animals are pumped with antibiotics to fight the inevitable infections they get from the unsanitary conditions. All of these hormones, medications, antibiotics, and viruses are in the food we ingest, subsequently making us inflamed and sick.

Pork is especially toxic, and the most cancer-promoting meat you can eat. Pigs are scavengers and harbor an enormous number of viruses, parasites, bacteria, and pathogens like worms, and hepatitis E. Also, pigs don't sweat due to not having any sweat glands. Therefore, pigs don't detox, and when we consume pig meat, we get all those pathogens and environmental toxins into our systems.

Wondering about ground turkey? In 2013, Consumer Reports investigated and reported that 69% of the ground turkey samples they tested harbored enterococcus and 60% harbored Escherichia coli. They also reported fecal contamination in many of the samples. Yikes.

The last form of meat I want to discuss is fish. Our oceans, lakes, and rivers are extremely hazardous. Our oceans are being polluted from waste from nuclear power plants and it's not getting any better. The waste materials include both liquids and solids housed in various containers, as well as reactor vessels, with nuclear fuel. So every time we eat fish, we subject ourselves to toxic waste. Shellfish are bottom feeders, eating and absorbing the toxins and pollution in the oceans, rivers, and lakes. When we eat fish and shellfish, we are exposed to the radioactive waste that accumulates in their tissues.

Tuna, shark, and swordfish eat a lot of the smaller fish and contain high levels of mercury. So we are not out of the woods if we decide to just eliminate the bottom feeders (scavengers) like shrimp, crab, lobster, catfish, and crawfish. These fish are all absorbing toxins from the environment.

The bottom line is, whether you are regularly eating factory-raised meat or fresh-caught fish, you are likely in a constant state of inflammation, which we know can lead to diseases like cancer, diabetes, heart disease, and more. When you have cancer, you cannot stress out your body with any animal meats.

Dairy

Dairy is also a huge concern when it comes to cancer growth due to its sugar, hormone and toxic contents. Most dairy products have over 60 different hormones in them, hormones that promote weight gain, estrogen dominance, leaky gut, and cancer growth. Dairy is not meant for human consumption; it is made for baby cows to become adult cows, so why are we drinking it? The other main reason is due to a genetically engineered bovine growth hormone (rbGH). Cows are treated with this growth hormone in order to increase the production of growth and milk. So you are getting rbGH in your milk, cheese, ice cream, and yogurt. Since the controversial approval of this drug in 1994 by the FDA, there have been substantial increases in lymphatic cancers.

Protein Powders — Oh, My?

Contrary to popular belief, most proteins are very toxic and cause inflammation in the body. When you have cancer it is important you understand why you should not be consuming protein drinks. First of all, as we discussed earlier with meat, protein will increase your IGF-1, and if you have cancer, you definitely do not want that to be elevated. Next, you have to know what kinds of proteins to avoid. Soy should absolutely be avoided. Soy is highly processed and contains enzyme inhibitors that turn off natural enzymes needed to perform critical cell functions, including blocking thyroid hormone. Any gluten-containing protein powders, like wheat, barley, rye etc., are highly allergenic and promote inflammation.

Whey protein powders made with whey from factory-raised cows contain the same antibiotics and hormones that we discussed earlier. The poor animals are not only pumped up with these drugs, but they are also being fed grains filled with pesticides and GMOs. Protein powders are also filled with unpronounceable fillers, food dyes, preservatives, hidden sugar, artificial sweeteners, and toxic oils such as canola and soy.

Chronic Inflammation

A new study by researchers at the Ohio State University Comprehensive Cancer Center — Arthur G. James Cancer Hospital and Richard J. Solove Research Institute (OSUCCC — James) found that inflammation can cause cancer. Chronic inflammation due to infection or to conditions such as chronic inflammatory bowel disease is associated with up to 25 percent of all cancers.

When a person is exposed to high amounts of toxins over time (many of which we discussed, like GMOs, meat, dairy, and environmental toxins), these toxins settle in your tissues. In Dr. Conner's book, *Stop Fighting Cancer and Start Treating the Cause*, he states that while most of the time you can't see or feel it, this low-grade, constant type of inflammation increases the risk of every leading cause of death. An inflammatory process starts when chemicals are released by the damaged tissue. Chronic inflammation may be caused by infections that don't go away, abnormal immune reactions to normal tissues, or conditions such as obesity. Over time, chronic inflammation can cause DNA damage and lead to cancer.

Just living in America these days exposed you to years of environmental toxins, dirty drinking water, and stressors that may lead to eating poorly, drinking, and drug abuse. The result is a suppressed immune system that makes it more difficult for your body to fight or kill off cancer. It is very common for someone with stiffness, arthritis, brain fog, and other chronic inflammatory symptoms to blame it on old age or, worse, allow the doctor to give them medications that might alleviate a symptom temporarily, but do not address or fix the underlying inflammation.

Bottom line: if you have cancer, you have inflammation. I did, and it surprised me that even being a functional diagnostic nutritionist and clean eater didn't exclude me from toxins and cancer. I had to learn what happened. What combination of things I could have been doing that caused my diagnosis. I learned so much, and a lot of what I learned, I am sharing with you in this book.

Action Steps

So now that we have discussed why sugar, GMOs, meat, and dairy are all promote cancer, let's talk about what good nutrition is and how it can heal your cancer. When you feed your body nutrient-dense foods from the earth, the nutrition will repair, rejuvenate, heal, and detoxify your body. Healthy foods from the earth will saturate your cells with powerful nutrients: enzymes, vitamins, minerals, and antioxidants that will destroy cancer and will support and build your immune system.

I understand what you must be thinking. What's left to eat? A lot, actually, and I can definitely help you with your options.

Eat only raw, organic fruits (in moderation) and vegetables. Yes, I said all raw and organic. Do it for a minimum of 90 days. When you eat whole raw fruits (not juiced) and vegetables, you are getting the maximum nutrition possible into your body, because the enzymes in the raw food make it very easy for your body to digest. Eating raw/organic will also build up your immune system to support apoptosis (the death of your cancer cells). The easiest way to cleanse your entire digestive system and get all the nutrients and fiber is to eat a lot of salads with an assortment of raw veggies. Add a little lemon juice or balsamic vinegar. The TOP anti-inflammatory and cancer fighting foods are dark green leafy vegetables like spinach, chard, collards, broccoli rabe, cabbage and kale and other foods like carrots, garlic, strawberries, tomatoes, cucumbers, onions, peppers, cauliflower, sprouts of all kinds, zucchini, squash, leeks, and asparagus. You want to make sure you have a lot of these foods. Raw preferably.

Blend and drink a vegetable smoothie every day. Note: I did not say juice, and I did not say a fruit smoothie. The difference between blending and juicing is this: blending liquefies all the ingredients, including pulp and fiber, for a smoothie that is nutrient-dense. Juicing, however, as with a fruit, means you're getting a lot of (natural) sugar and no fiber. I drank a 32-ounce blended vegetable smoothie every single day, packed with over a dozen different vegetables, fruit, and other ingredients. I did *not* juice, ever. I didn't want to drink fruit that was juiced, mainly because I didn't want my blood sugar to spike, and I also didn't think juicing would keep me satisfied. I know a lot of cancer patients who juice, which is fine. I did not. I drank one giant green smoothie per day, and then ate a lot of raw organic salads and vegetables the rest of the day. If you go to www.irefusedchemorecipes.com you can download my favorite cancer-fighting smoothie.

Follow the Budwig Protocol and eat quark. There is one nutritional therapeutic protocol that I used during my healing of lymphoma, and I am a strong believer in this mixture. Dr. Johanna Budwig, a German biochemist, was researching the pathogenesis of disease and illness and discovered that quark (any soft, fresh, organic, low-fat cottage cheese) contained the very same sulphydryl groups found in cancer treatment drugs. She also discovered that PUFAs (polyunsaturated fatty acids) are major components of cellular membranes critical to energy. She found that by mixing cottage cheese and flax oil (which is a PUFA), a chemical reaction took place when the sulphydryl groups in the cheese bound with the unsaturated fatty acids in the flaxseed oil, allowing it to enter the cells and supply energy. The short explanation: when Dr. Budwig gave her cancer patients quark and flax oil, her patients had improved oxygen supply to their cells, and many were healed. You see, cancer cells, unlike normal healthy cells, do not like oxygen, using sugar instead for growth. You want to get as much oxygen to your cells as possible, to starve the cancer.

Your nutrition and what you eat must be the *very* first thing you change. I put all of my clients on very specific nutrition protocols that, first and foremost, start to repair their immune function. In my REFUSED Solution program, I give them tons of recipes, smoothie combinations, and cooking ideas.

I understand the overwhelm you feel when you try to figure out where to start. I will help you with that. I have a very simple yet effective nutrition protocol that will get you started on your way. My clients always feel so much more at ease knowing that they are being coached throughout the entire process. They don't have to figure out all of this by themselves. Our goal is to help you with your overwhelm. The food you put in your body is key, and it's the first thing you need to change. It is true that food is our medicine, and medicine is our food.

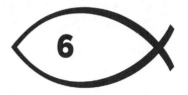

6

U — UNITING WITH GOD

*I sought the Lord and he answered me and
delivered me from all my fears.*

– Psalm 34:4

A few days after my cancer diagnosis, a girlfriend and I were talking and crying over my situation. She was so sad and worried for me. She said that she just didn't understand why God would allow this to happen to me: a woman who is always trying to help others; who does good in her own life; and who has worked hard to take care of her physical self. I often asked myself that question, too. Why would God allow this to happen to me? How can this happen when I have been committed to honoring God in the area of my health? I have never been one to abuse my body. I don't drink, smoke, or eat crap. I rarely ever take over-the-counter medications. I've devoted my life to really taking care of my body, or so I thought. So when I got the news of cancer, this was a struggle for me. I was angry, confused, frustrated, and hurt.

You see, I am a Christian. A Christian is not about following a certain religion, or what church or group you affiliate yourself with. It is about having a relationship with God and believing in the Bible. The Bible is my life's guidebook. There is an answer for every single struggle you have in life, in the Bible. So when I got diagnosed with cancer, although I didn't like it and it felt a bit like a slap in the face, I had to go to my Father and read my Bible for help. There was just no way I could have handled something this big by myself. No way. This was a life-and-death situation I was facing. The only way I knew how to cope was to ask God, pray, and have Him guide me in what to do. So that's what I did.

After my diagnosis, I was devastated, angry, confused, scared, upset, and I couldn't even pray. I didn't know what to say. My initial thought was, "Really? All I have done my entire life is to try to serve You, honor You, and take care of my body, and this is what I get?" I'm not going to lie, that first couple days after I was diagnosed was a complete mental break down. I wanted to quit. I was like, "What's the point?"

My selfish side was saying: I don't want to be sick and live life with being sick. My ego side was saying: I don't want to lose my hair and be seen as the sickly fitness guru. My human side was saying: this is too much for me to handle; I won't do this. I can't do this! And I was right. I could *not* do this alone. I had to go to the only one that I know could help me.

You see, God has never, ever failed me. Even though I have been a Christian all of my life, I have had many traumatic life experiences. God has never let me down, and what I mean by that is that in every single situation in my life that was traumatic, He always, 100% of the time, turned the situation into a positive and I was better for it.

Situation: I went through a divorce. It was horrible, stressful, and embarrassing.

Result: God led me to Mark, my rock, and he is my life's biggest blessing.

Situation: I was suddenly laid off from my corporate job, eliminating my income overnight. I had no idea how I was going to support myself financially.

Result: God opened doors for me in my fitness and health career path. I would never have pursued my passion for health and fitness if I hadn't been laid off.

Situation: After a year of trying to figure out what was going on, I found out I had adrenal fatigue. I had been feeling really bad. I'd gained a lot of weight (despite my healthy eating and working out), I was very fatigued, and my faith was being tested.

Result: I learned a lot about the body, and that led me to become a holistic functional diagnostic nutritionist and hormone coach. I have helped hundreds of women in a totally different way.

Situation: A business investor tried to hostilely overtake our business venture with numerous other business partners.

Result: He didn't win. The courts saw through his scheme, and their ruling led me to be able to get rid of the toxic business partners and move forward with my dream of owning a studio and consulting business.

Situation: I lost a lease for my business and was told I had two weeks to find a new facility and move my entire gym and clients. I thought I was done!

Result: God provided a perfect location only three miles from the old one, and I wasn't closed for a single day (except to move). It was an amazing turn of events that could have only been orchestrated by God.

Situation: I tore my ACL during one of my women's fitness events. I was extremely stressed out and worried about the outcome of having surgery.

Result: I was forced to take some much-needed mental and physical time off and ended up not having to have surgery. God gave me new empathy for those with injuries. I learned to rehab my knee myself, avoiding any surgery at all, and my knee is doing great to this day.

Situation: I had a fallout with a dear friend that caused extreme stress and emotional trauma. During this period of time, I felt my health really took a turn for the worse.

Result: God healed this friendship, and she and I became better friends. I was able to let go of the horrible resentment, anger, and hurt … only God could do this for me. I learned that having tension in relationships definitely causes physical symptoms, and is not something God wants us to have in our lives.

Situation: CANCER — this was my life's biggest challenge to this day. It was a wakeup call for my health, quality of life, and relationship with God.

Result: I can honestly say that cancer *changed me*. It taught me lessons that I would never, ever have learned if I hadn't gone through this journey. God taught me so much about faith, fear, worry, love, compassion, and also physiology. God was the only way I knew how to handle this crisis. I had to give this entire life situation over to the one who has *never* failed me, my gracious and loving heavenly Father.

The other amazing thing that cancer has created for me, is a renewal of my passion for helping others. I now serve with a stronger conviction and a servant's heart. Cancer broke me, but to only build me up stronger than ever. I will be even stronger for my clients. I will be healthier for my clients. I will serve them better than ever. This is my desire. To be there for you, my dear reader. To be there for you, to help you get through your tough time. I understand. I've been there. I can help you!

After my weekend of despair, anger, sadness, fear, and panic. I sat down and prayed. I mean, really prayed. I prayed to God, asking Him for help. I was incapable of handling this myself. I didn't even know where to begin, where to start. Immediately after I pleaded with Him, saying that prayer, He led me to scripture. I read the Bible because I know that when God leads me to a scripture, it is Him talking to me. When God leads me to scripture, it might be through a sermon at church, through a devotion that I read that day, or a verse from a dear friend. Sometimes, when I am praying, a verse or idea will pop into my mind to read. These are all ways I know God is leading me.

In an excerpt from my journal, dated March 21st, I wrote down the scriptures to which I'd been led:

> *"I have told you these things, so that in me, you may have peace. In this world you will have trouble. But take heart! I have overcome the world."*
>
> – John 16:33

I was being told that in spite of the inevitable struggles in the world that I will face, I will not be alone. Jesus does not abandon us to our struggles. If we remember this, our ultimate victory has already been won. We can claim the peace of Christ in the most troublesome times. We don't have to let worry be a part of our struggles. He has given us courage, confidence, assurance, and peace.

I was also led to these:

> *"Come to me, all you who are heavy laden,*
> *and I will give you rest."*
>
> – Matthew 11: 28

> *"The Lord will fight for you, all you have to*
> *do is be still."*
>
> – Exodus 14: 14

Wow, this hit home. God was telling me at that moment that I can have peace in Him and go to Him, and He will give me rest. He is going to fight for me. These scriptures instantly spoke to me. They were a direct word coming from my Father. Now I just had to listen and do.

This was my prayer, which I also wrote in my journal after reading and studying these scriptures:

> *"I thank you Father — that my life is a journey. I am not going to stay stuck in a difficult or trying situation forever. You are taking me through it. Help me to experience our joys regardless of my situation. I know you are with me. I ask you to guide me. Guide my path, show me, and reveal to me how you want me to handle this*

situation. I have no clue what to do next. I trust you —
I love you — I worship you — I need you. Please make
my decision for me right now. Make them so clear to me
and reveal to me your guiding presence. AMEN."

After studying His word, hearing His voice and praying this prayer, I instantly had peace. Instantly! You see, when you pray, you are talking to God. You are communicating with Him. It's like having a conversation with your best friend. That is what praying is. It's a conversation. So when I pray and I read my Bible, I am communicating with my friend. How I hear back from Him is through scripture and through my spiritual guided intuition.

This is truly the only way that I was able to get through my cancer crisis. I had to put my faith, trust, and entire life into my Father's hand. He spoke back, He revealed Himself to me on numerous occasions ... this is what He does when you take that step of faith and reach out to get to know Him. He will NOT reach out to you unless you are a willing participant. It's no different than a friendship. Think of your closest friends. Do you talk with them daily? Do you have a mutual respect, honesty, and openness with them? This is how God works. You can't expect Him to reveal Himself to you, or help you, if it's one-sided. God was my counselor, my leader, the director in my life. Not only during my cancer scare, but in everything else in life. This is the only way I can get through what comes at me.

That day and the next few days, I had instant courage to fight for what I felt God wanted me to do. That meant, I was going to find answers on how to go about curing my cancer without chemo or radiation. I'd never had peace about going that direction, anyway. I had to listen to my inner voice, because I strongly believe that inner voice (intuition) is another way God speaks to me. When I have an intuition about something, I am usually always right. I don't say this to brag, I say it because I really try to be in tune with what God tells me. I pray for this almost every day. My intuition (very strong sense) about not doing chemo and radiation, was pretty solid. When I started researching, all the information I was needed to confirm my decision fell into my lap. I found a woman who had the same type of cancer that I did, and I was able to learn from her what she did and how she healed herself. I instantly found books, DVDs, and articles. I spent hours, days, and many sleepless nights reading, watching videos, and talking to people.

Initially, Mark was under the assumption that chemo and radiation were my only options, and at first, he strongly encouraged traditional treatment. He just didn't know, and neither did I, really. The only thing I knew at the time was that I didn't have peace about undergoing those harmful treatments. But when I told him I was going to refuse chemo and radiation and that I needed him to be my researcher so we could learn everything we could about cancer, he said, "Ok, I'm on it." He literally took a leave of absence from the job he was doing at that time and became a full-time cancer researcher.

My husband … can I just say what an amazing man he is? I truly am so very proud to call this man my husband. He is a man of God, and his faith was an amazing help to me. He was right by my side, praying for me, helping me, and supporting me with everything in regard to my emotions and health. I know this was not easy for him, being on the other side of illness. He has shared with me that seeing me go through this was extremely hard on him, and at times he didn't know what to do, so he prayed.

He got answers like I did when I prayed. We got answers... we became prayer warriors. It was the only way we got through. We called ourselves TEAM DALE, because we were indeed a team, fighting the biggest battle of our lives.

There would be times when he would research or read something and tell me that I needed to do something, eat something, supplement with something — I mean, every day we would learn something new. I recall one time when I was at my office, and I knew he was at home studying, and I called him and asked him, "So, what supplement am I going to be trying next?" We also had to make it a priority to work on my stress, so we would practice "laugh therapy," which is one thing Mark does very well. He makes me laugh. He is so witty and funny. After 13 years of marriage, he still giggles like a giddy school girl.

He was amazing. I still had to run my business, which meant mentoring clients, doing the financials, managing employees, running camps, giving presentations, teaching classes, and creating programs. It also took a lot of time to prep food, shop for all the organic supplies, and undergo all of my holistic treatments. I also had to try and find as much time as I could to study and research. Mark did most of the research, initially. It was so great to have someone fully committed to and supportive of my decision. My parents were also on board, but not at first. They were frightened of the unknown, scared for their daughter, and didn't know about the holistic options available. The cancer world does not condone, approve, or recognize holistic alternative treatments. So I asked my parents to read a couple of books that I found super helpful and informative, so that they would understand why I was so adamant about healing my body with natural protocols. Once they read a few of the materials, they, too, became more at peace with my decision and were very supportive.

A few days later, on March 24, I received more from God during my devotional time. It was about the criteria for making important decisions. Again, this was just another confirmation that the decision I was making to REFUSE chemo was in line with what God wanted me to do. I wrote it down in my journal:

I. *Acts 1:21–25 — God tells us to do three things when making a big decision:*

1. *Set up criteria consistent with the Bible*

2. *Examine the alternatives*

3. *Pray for wisdom and guidance to reach a wise decision*

If anyone of you lacks wisdom, he should ask God, who gives generously without fault and it will be given to him.

– James 1:5

By wisdom, James is talking not only about knowledge but about the ability to make wise decision in difficult times/circumstances. Whenever we need wisdom, we can pray to God and He will generously supply what we need. To learn God's will, we need to read His word and ask Him to show us how to obey it and then we must do what He tells us.

This was my Word from God on March 24th, after studying this scripture and praying for wisdom:

"'You are doing the right thing, you are on the right path. Keep your eyes focused on me and let me fight this battle. I

love you, Teri. I will lead and protect and heal you.' Tears!
Thank you, Jesus, for speaking these words to me."

The next few weeks, of course, were an emotional roller coaster. Although I never once questioned my decision to fight this holistically, I was faced a lot with fear and worry.

I'm human, and of course worry is my Everest. But God is very clear in the Bible that we are not to worry. I have been a worrier all of my life, and I think God was finally trying to get through to me, wake me up with cancer to tell me this. QUIT WORRYING! Your worry is causing you too much stress in your life, and what for? *Matthew 6:34* says, "Do not worry or be anxious about tomorrow, for tomorrow will have worries and anxieties of its own."

> I Peter 5:7 — Cast all your cares on Him, because He cares for you.
>
> Psalm 56:3 — When I am afraid, I put my trust in you.
>
> Phil 4:6-7 — Do not be anxious about anything, but in everything by prayer and supplication with thanksgiving let your requests be made known to God. And the peace of God, which surpasses all understanding, will guard your hearts and your minds in Christ Jesus.
>
> Isaiah 41:10 — Fear not, (there is nothing to fear) for I am with you.

More than any other command in scripture, God tells us not to fear 365 times. Isn't it interesting that it turns out that "fear not" appears 365 times, one for every day of the year? Hmmm … must be a reason why this is such a powerful reminder. God didn't intend for Christians to spend their days preoccupied with anxiety and worry. I love what Pastor Rick Warren says about why fear is mentioned 365 times in the Bible: "Why did God stress the importance of avoiding fear? Because our hurts and hang-ups can often cause us to think that God is out to get us, that all He wants to do is condemn us and punish us. But that simply isn't true. Jesus is the proof of that."

When Christians form a healthy relationship with God and understand His eternal grace and mercy, they will realize that there is no real need for fear. God isn't trying to get even with you. Jesus has taken the penalty for everything you've ever done wrong or will do wrong. He paid for it on the cross. This is why I put my faith in God and have to daily remind myself that I am not allowed to worry and have fear. There is no point. God is in control and is not going to let me down. You see, when you have faith, then you don't worry.

Faith: My Life's Verse (Phil 4:13)

"I can do all things through Christ who strengthens me."

– Phil 4:13

Why do I choose faith? First and foremost, I believe there is a God because of my relationship with Him. He is real, He has spoken to me, led me, and guided me through many horrible events in my life. Faith is released by praying, saying, and doing whatever God asks me to do. It's really that simple. Faith is a mindset. This kind of faith is a relationship that expects God to act. When we act on this with expectation, we can overcome our fears. We need to let God deal with our fears and just trust Him. This is the antidote for fear.

> *Hebrews 11:1 — Now Faith is the assurance of things hope for, the conviction of things not seen.*
>
> *Hebrews 11:6 — and without faith it is impossible to please God, because anyone who come to him must believe that he exists and that he rewards those who earnestly seek him. Faith unlocks the promises of God. Faith gives us the power to hold on in rough times. Faith teaches us lessons only to help us grow. Faith doesn't always take you out of a problem, it takes you through it and gives you the ability to handle the pain. Faith doesn't always take you out of the storm, it calms you in the midst of the storm.*
>
> *Matthew 21:22 — If you believe, you will receive whatever you ask for in prayer*
>
> *1 Thessalonians 5:17 — Pray without ceasing.*
>
> *John 14:14 — You may ask me for anything in my name and I will do it.*

Faith was a huge part of me getting well. Having a cancer diagnosis causes so much emotional stress, and letting it go and giving it to God takes away the worry and the fear. I kept these verses with me at all times. I printed out eight pages of scripture verses to have on hand, so that anytime I was stricken with worry, fear, or doubt, I could read these verses, over and over. I would also always remind myself that God has *never* failed me. He has turned every storm, battle, and crisis in my life into something good. This is what I knew to be true of my cancer journey. I knew He would turn this into something good.

I encourage you, my dear friend, to read the Bible. Pray for wisdom, pray for direction, pray for God to reveal Himself to you. God promised to reveal Himself to you if you step out in faith and seek Him. He will give you what you need to go through this battle. I have been praying over this book since day one of writing it, hoping that it serves as a way to encourage, lead, and direct you to the answers that are best for you. I promise you this: going through cancer will be better with God than without Him. My love for you in writing this book is to tell you this truth.

It is also important that you find someone in your life who will support you in your decision and educate themselves right alongside of you. Tell them to read this book. If you have someone in your life who will stand beside you, help you research, and go through the process with you, it will help you.

God often allows crisis in our lives in order to get our attention. When we get flattened, flat on our backs, we are forced to look up. Do you feel like you have been nudged to look up? I believe that by reading this book, God is trying to speak to you. He wants you to seek Him. Look up. This will be your source of strength, peace, comfort, and healing.

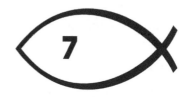

S — SUPPLEMENTS

*"A control for cancer is known, and it comes
from nature, but it is not widely available to
the public because it cannot be patented,
and therefore is not commercially attractive
to the pharmaceutical industry."*

– G. Edward Griffin

One of my very first experiences with supplements was back years ago when I was working in corporate America. I was struggling, struggling, struggling for energy. I kept long hours and had a very stressful job in telecommunications. I would wake up at 4:00 am, get to the gym by 5:00 am to work out, and then commute in bad traffic to my corporate job and be stressed out all day in a very demanding position. In the evenings, I taught aerobics classes, and I was just starting to get in the fitness industry. I wouldn't get home until 9 or 10 at night. I was putting in long hours and I was exhausted, so I had a habit of drinking a lot of coffee. I mean a *lot*. In fact, I would go to Super America gas station (SA) after my morning workout and sip on coffee during my long commute to the office. I would get those huge, 32 oz. cups and I would add the sugary cappuccino flavoring the SA store had ... yum, it was good.

I needed the caffeine to keep me awake for the job, and I wanted the sugar because I had so many cravings for sweet things. Then, around lunchtime, I would go to Super America (SA) gas station again, and get another coffee to get me through the afternoon, then on my commute home and before I taught classes at night I would drink another cup of SA coffee. I was addicted. I drank so much hot coffee for energy that my gums were hurting. Sometimes they would even bleed. Plus, I would crash a couple of hours after I drank coffee, and it was bad. This is why I kept having to drink it throughout the day. The instant buzz was great, but the crash was awful and the side effects of all that caffeine were not good. I had stomach aches besides the bleeding gums. Ironically, I didn't have vibrant steady energy all day long, although that's what I thought the coffee would give me.

A girlfriend of mine at the time had been after me to come to one of her supplement meetings. She was heavily into supplements, but back then I was not a believer in supplements at all. In fact, I didn't know much about them, so I thought they were a scam and a waste of money. But my girlfriend was persistent in trying to educate me, because she knew my habitual coffee habits, and I was always complaining to her about my energy and gut aches. She insisted I come to one of her supplement seminars. So I gave in and went. I sat in the back of the room with my arms crossed. I'm sure I was giving off a very disinterested attitude, but I really didn't want to be there. They started the seminar off by passing around a drink for us to try. It tasted like Kool Aid. Pretty good. About a half-hour into the seminar, she asked all of us if we felt anything from the drink we'd consumed. I did not. Of course I didn't, because I was not a believer. I was going to prove to her that her supplements were a gimmick. Ha. Then she said this:

"So, the drink I gave everyone is a vitamin B drink with a unique blend of 20 vitamins and nutrients that are synergistically working together to provide a healthy source of energy, mental focus, and alertness. You should feel something after drinking this, not a shaky type of feeling, but like a burst of mental energy and focus."

I was like: yeah, right. I felt nothing. But then she went on to say, "If you do *not* feel this, then you are *not* absorbing nutrients. This vitamin drink is so effective at getting into your system that if you are not feeling something, it means you are toxic and your body is not absorbing the nutrients."

Hmmm…. This actually made sense to me. She went on to say that when a person is toxic, they don't feel the best and get cravings for sugar. This was me! I decided to try some of these supplements to see if I would start feeling better.

The next week, I did a detox supplement. I seriously was blown away. I honestly couldn't believe how well this detox supplement worked, because when I drank that same energy drink a few days later, I felt it working — big-time. My body was responded to these supplements. I started drinking that vitamin/energy drink, and I instantly no longer had the desire for my SA coffees. This was unbelievable to me! I'd craved those SA coffees with a vengeance. To not crave coffee and sugar after only a couple weeks of using these supplements? I was impressed. I no longer crashed throughout the day, my stomach aches were gone, and so was the bleeding in my gums. It's been 25 years, and to this day, I have not had those cravings nor the need for the SA coffees. I still drink the vitamin drink a few times a week. It's a treat.

This started my quest for learning about supplements. What are they? Are they safe? Do they work? Can they take the place of medications?

A dietary supplement is a product intended for ingestion that contains an ingredient that will add further value to a normal diet. A dietary ingredient would be a substance like a vitamin, mineral, herb, botanical, amino acid, or an extract. Most dietary supplements are ingredients that are in nature. Dietary supplements may be found in a capsule, soft gel, liquid, powder, or tablet. They can ensure that you get an adequate dietary intake of essential nutrients that you either lack or need to increase. In addition, they can help reduce your risk of disease or heal your disease.

It is important to understand the difference between a supplement and a medication. So many people think supplements are a scam, like I used to until I started to learn and really understand what they are and how they work. You see, supplements are ingredients that your body recognizes as nutrition. Your body will recognize the ingredient and then utilize it in the body for purposes of health and healing. A medication is synthetic (man-made from a lab), and is not found in nature. Medications are a substance used for medical treatment to treat a condition or symptom. Your body does not recognize it as a vitamin, mineral, or healthy substance, it considers it a toxin in the body. Although the medication will sometimes treat the symptom, it doesn't cure or fix the health problem. It's like a bandage to cover up the symptom temporarily. More times than not, the medication will create a new symptom due to its toxic properties. Remember, modern doctors are taught virtually nothing about nutrition, nor do they study what makes the body healthy. They study disease and how to medicate that disease with synthetic drugs. I know this first hand because I went down the traditional medical path first. I had to understand what my options were. I went to two medical doctors, one ear, nose, and throat specialist, two oncologists and spoke with numerous PA's and specialists. They all told me that chemo and radiation were the best options and the only options that they knew of. This did not sit well with me and so that's when I decided to dig deep and figure out other options.

Here are some supplements I used as well as a few that I think anyone diagnosed with cancer could definitely start. There is a lot of scientific research out there on certain compounds in supplements proving to have significant anti-cancer effects. But if you have a "quick fix" mentality when it comes to supplements, you are missing the mark. First and foremost, you must douse your body with high quality nutrition/food first. Then add additional resources to make sure you are giving your body the maximum amount of healing power.

We've been told by pharmaceutical companies and the doctors who prescribe medications that there is an "instant fix" via pills for everything. And so sometimes people are tempted to believe that taking a bunch of supplements and not cleaning up one's nutrition will work. Not so. I healed my cancer by doing everything in my power to boost my own immune system. It takes time to reverse the damage that was already done, and there is a combination of things you must do, there is just not one single supplement or one best way. It just does not work like that. With all this being said, here is my top list of supplements that I used and I had great success with.

Starting Supplements

Artemisinin — Artemisinin is a substance derived from the leaves of a sweet wormwood plant known as artemisia annual. Artemisinin is a chemical compound that reacts with iron to form free radicals that can selectively destroy cancer cells from within while leaving normal cells untouched and unharmed. Many studies from the University of California and University of Washington found that artemisinin can stop the proliferation or multiplication of prostate cancer cells by arresting the cell cycle at a certain point. Researchers also looked into the effect of artemisinin on breast cancer cells. They found that artemisinin also caused an arrest at a certain point in the cell cycle of the cancer cells, thus disrupting the responsiveness of cancer cells to the hormone estrogen.

Apple Cider Vinegar — ACV has numerous health benefits like stabilizing blood sugar, killing bacteria, supplying energy, supporting metabolism, treating acid reflux, promoting alkalinity, neutralizing hormones, improving cholesterol levels, and more. The main reason I took it was to detoxify my lymphatic system. The antioxidants found in ACV reduce oxidative damage done to the body by free radicals. ACV improves the health of our blood and organs.

Beta Glucan — Beta glucan is a polysaccharide that is an immunomodulator, which means it activates and enhances your immune response to invaders like bacteria, viruses, and cancer. Beta glucans also stimulate the assembly of the immune stem cells inside bone marrow and supercharge immune cells to recognize complementary immune defense compounds. The research supports the ability of beta glucans to reduce the growth rate of cancer cells all while stimulating a stronger immune response to foreign invaders. **Research also shows that this may even be a stronger therapy than chemotherapy or radiation**, with no adverse health reactions. Beta glucans do not naturally occur within the body and need to be consumed from sources such as mushrooms and yeast. They come in capsule form.

Curcumin — One of the most important nutrients for cancer, curcumin is the yellow pigment that is extracted from turmeric. Over 2000 published studies have shown that curcumin has successfully combated many kinds of cancer. Curcumin actually stops cancer cells from dividing and triggers apoptosis (cell death). There have been many clinical trials proving its efficacy as an anti-cancer modality, but curcumin is not prescribed in cancer therapy because there is no financial incentive to do so. Drug companies cannot patent natural substances, like any that I have listed so far. Without a patent, there is no profit. Not only is it the top supplement for cancer, but it is tremendously effective in reducing inflammation and chronic pain and is of great benefit in treating autoimmune disorders, heart health, and depression. I can't say enough positive things about the health benefits of curcumin.

Vitamin D3 — Vitamin D really isn't a vitamin; it's actually considered a hormone, because it gets converted into a steroid hormone that regulates well over 1,000 different physiological processes and controls around five percent of the human genome (DNA). You primarily get Vitamin D from the sun. When the sun's ultraviolet B ("UVB") rays hit your skin, they trigger a pre-cholesterol molecule (7-dehydrocholesterol), which is then turned into Vitamin D3 (aka cholecalciferol). The mechanisms by which vitamin D reduces the risk of cancer are fairly well understood. They include enhancing calcium absorption, inducing cell differentiation, increasing apoptosis (programmed cell death), reducing metastasis and proliferation, and reducing angiogenesis (formation of new blood vessels). It is critical for cancer patients to have adequate Vitamin D. It also squelches cancer at a genetic level. Vitamin D deficiency is directly linked to cancer. My Vitamin D levels were so low, that my body was not functioning normally or performing apoptosis. In order to heal your cancer, your Vitamin D blood levels should be higher than the standard levels.

B17/Laetrile — B17, otherwise known as laetrile, is very easy to find in nature, but it is very complex to explain how it works killing cancer. The abbreviated explanation is that there is a process in the body and a certain way that laetrile unlocks the enzyme found in cancer cells and opens it up to create a targeted poison that kills the cancer cell. It's kind of like "natural chemo." If you really want to understand the science, the research is readily available. I've chosen to simplify it for myself and others, so my clients don't feel overwhelmed. You can find B17/laetrile in apricot seeds. You want to know something really shocking, though? I learned this from Dr. Conners, who told me, "The FDA has made the purchase of laetrile supplements very difficult to obtain, even though it is a very safe and natural supplement to take. In order for a doctor to use laetrile, they must have a patient sign a statement that the treatment is solely for detoxification and NOT to cure cancer. In other words, all 'treatment for cancer,' not just laetrile, is effectively illegal unless one is an oncologist." Amazing, huh? You can purchase apricot seeds online or get them at your local organic store. They are very bitter tasting, but I didn't mind them. I ate them every day and I still eat them today.

Essiac Tea — Essiac tea is an ancient recipe that originated with the Ojibwe tribes of Native Americans. It has been around and utilized for years, and is known as the "Ojibwe Tea of Life." It is a powerful and effective natural cancer treatment. Again, it has been scrutinized by the medical mainstream because it is an herbal supplement that can't be patented. Essiac tea is made up of four herbs: burdock root, slippery elm, sheep sorrel, and Indian rhubarb root. A Canadian nurse, Rene Caisse (Essiac is "Caisse" spelled backwards), was the first to use it during the 1920s to help her patients who were suffering from various forms of cancer, and many of them were healed. Thousands of patient testimonials led to the popularity of Essiac tea, and it can still be found in health stores today. These herbs are very powerful for immune support. They destroy bad bacteria, viruses, and parasites, and detoxify the colon, liver, and kidneys. The antioxidant cocktail in Essiac tea is also a potent defense against free radicals. I drank it every day for about six months on my protocol.

Matcha Green Tea — Oh, Matcha, how I love thee. This is my absolute favorite discovery that I used every day on my anti-cancer protocol. I still drink this every single day. It has so many amazing health benefits. Matcha is a special type of powdered green tea that is grown and produced in Japan. There is a very special process that takes place when growing the leaves. Matcha leaves are packed with chlorophyll, and the leaves are carefully ground to produce a fine green powder. Do not confuse Matcha with green tea that you can steep and purchase in bags. Matcha has very high concentrations of antioxidants like polyphenols and EGCG (100 times more than regular green tea). Matcha increases energy, boosts antioxidants and metabolism, and is excellent for heart, brain, and skin health. Matcha delivers mega-doses of cancer-fighting EGCG, which is an antioxidant only found in green tea.

Medicinal Mushrooms — I had never heard of mushrooms as a supplement before, but I quickly understood the importance of them when I was diagnosed with cancer and wanted to stimulate my immune system into fighting and finding circulating tumor cells. What I learned was that mushrooms contain many chemicals, antioxidants, immune modulators, polysaccharides and more that all play an important role in attacking cancerous cells, detoxifying, improving oxygen utilization, improving liver function, and strengthening the body's immune system functions. They are also potent antioxidant free-radical scavengers. It's important to take a variety of mushrooms, like Cordyceps, Agaricus, Reishi, and Maitake. (Note: I am not referring to hallucinogenic Psilocybin mushrooms.) Dr. Conners has a special dry mushroom blend that I drank every day and still do. Understanding the importance of how these play a role in fighting and preventing cancer will help you when you drink it down. Looks like mud, but I figured out a way to make it so it wasn't too bad. It looks way worse than it tastes.

Chlorella — Chlorella is extremely nutrient-dense. It is a fresh water algae that promotes detoxification, and is packed with vitamin C, minerals, amino acids, essential fatty acids, phytonutrients, zinc, GLA, and chlorophyll. Not only does it play a huge role in detoxifying the body, but it also promotes healthy cell membranes and insulin receptor sites. Chlorella is known as a heavy metals detoxifier, and is also known to help pull out toxins from the body that have bio toxins from tuberculosis, Lyme disease, tetanus, and mold. It's been said to cleanse the blood, digestive tract, and liver. Chlorella also has the ability to protect against inflammation and infection, as well as lower blood pressure and cholesterol levels. In cancer, it inhibits cancer cell activity and the development of malignant activity. It has been proven to suppress the new generation of blood vessels required by cancer cells in order to grow. So many incredible benefits. I added one teaspoon a day to my green smoothie.

Spirulina — Spirulina is a blue-green algae. It is full of antioxidants, vitamins, minerals, protein, and carotenoids. It is superfood that helps protect your cells from damage. Spirulina is a great source of B vitamins, calcium, beta carotene, and iron, and also contains healthy fats like GLA, EPA, DHA, and ALA. It is an anti-inflammatory. Cancer in the body will metastasize when cancer stem cells are not killed in the body. Spirulina is one of the super phytonutrients that targets cancer stem cells and eliminates tumors. I put one teaspoon a day in my green smoothie.

Wheat Grass — Wheat grass is an edible, gluten-free grass that is either milled down into a fine green powder or juiced into a "wheat grass" shot. It is packed with important nutrients. It is known as a "superfood," and is loaded with amino acids, enzymes needed for digestion, and many vitamins and minerals. Some of the important benefits: it helps oxygenate the body, alkalinizes the body, is full of chlorophyll and iron, rebuilds blood, boosts metabolism, purifies liver, reduces inflammation, improves digestion, detoxifies the body of heavy metals, and helps regulate blood sugar. This whole food demonstrates enormous anti-cancer potential, in that it seems to do so through the mechanism of inducing apoptosis (which is the death of cancerous cells). With all the benefits that this little guy has, why not have it a part of your supplement schedule?

Citrus Pectin — Citrus pectin is an important supplement that everyone with cancer should consider. As you know, circulating tumor cells (CTCs) in the bloodstream eventually latch on to the lining of blood vessel walls for the process of metastasis to start. But what if the cancer cells couldn't latch onto the blood vessel wall? What if they would just continue to wander through the blood stream, incapable of forming metastases? This would allow our immune system (white blood cells) to find the CTCs and kill them. This is, in essence, what citrus pectin does. Normally, citrus pectin is very hard for the body to absorb, but scientists have figured out a way to modify it so that it is absorbed into the blood stream, where it halts the growth of new cancer cells and stops the CTCs from attaching to the blood vessel wall, reducing the cancer aggressiveness and metastasis. Pretty amazing, huh? There's a lot of science behind this powerful little cancer killer, and it's also inexpensive and very safe. Why wouldn't every person with cancer want to be on this? I took one teaspoon a day in my smoothie.

Amla Powder — Amla, also known as Indian gooseberry, is probably one of the most powerful antioxidants in the world. It is also one of the world's best-known sources of vitamin C. It is rich in fiber and chromium, and is known to help reduce risk of cancer, especially in the gastrointestinal and respiratory tract. This is a very potent anti-cancer superfood.

Flaxseed — Flaxseed, another cancer-fighting food, is an ideal source of fiber, omega-3 fat, and lignan. Lignan has been known to reduce the size of cancerous tumors in research labs. *The Journal of Clinical Cancer Research* published a study that showed that flaxseed may decrease the risk of breast cancer, and

The Journal of Nutrition published a study showing that lignan reduces the risk of endometrial and ovarian cancers.

Frankincense — Frankincense and its potential to fight cancer is a highly controversial topic in the research world. I did decide to use it due to its anti-inflammatory properties; specifically, frankincense has been shown to be a potent inhibitor of 5-lipoxygenase, an enzyme responsible for inflammation in the body. It also helps boost immune function, improves circulation, and aids in digestion. There is current research that demonstrates anti-mutagenic and apoptotic properties in many cancer studies. I remember watching an interview with a girl who had a brain stem tumor. She had surgery to remove the tumor, but they were only successful in removing half of the tumor. She said she was doing an all-organic diet along with the frankincense oil, also known as "liquid gold." Every couple of hours, she put a drop of frankincense on her tongue and pressed it up against the roof of her mouth. She continued this protocol, and in three years, her tumor was gone. She and her doctor attribute her recovery to frankincense and her nutrition protocol.

Remember, that none of the above alternative holistic supplements will ever be able to be prescribed in cancer therapy, because there is no financial incentive to do so. Drug companies cannot patent natural substances. Without a patent there is no profit. Sad, annoying, and frustrating — but true. This is why we must do our own research and be our own health detectives. Also, all of these supplements are non-toxic. You don't need a prescription, you just need to drive to your local organic health store, where you will be able to find most of these items. That doesn't mean that you should go out and buy every single supplement and start taking it. You must do your due diligence.

WORD OF CAUTION: If you start to take a supplement and are also on medications, there could be contraindications to the particular treatment. So you must be careful and always check with your physician before starting any supplements.

The last thing I want to say is this. Although I strongly believe that the supplements discussed in this chapter worked for me, it is impossible to know which ones helped me and which ones didn't. I am quite certain that some might have been a waste of money, but I didn't have any side effects from any of the above, I felt absolutely fantastic the entire time I was fighting my lymphoma, and none of these were toxic, like chemo and radiation. I wasn't afraid to take the supplements, and every single one was worth trying. Again, I really had to use common sense and how I felt as well as measuring the progress of my healing in my decision to try them, stay on them, and go off some of them.

My entire cancer journey was really learning and understanding my body and how it worked. Really listening to it and at the same time providing it with the highest quality nutrition and supplementation that I could. This was my mission. Now, it's my mission to help *you*! In the REFUSED Solution Program, I am able to make suggestions for you on high-quality supplements that are proven to help with fighting cancer and inflammation.

I'm guessing that now that you've read this chapter, you're feeling a little overwhelmed and uncertain of where to start. This is normal. Not everyone will need all of these supplements when healing their cancer; everyone is different. The good news is that I can help take the confusion out of where to start and what to take. Some very common feedback I get from my clients is that they love the fact that I help them sort through all the information. They don't have to feel stressed and pressured to try things that they are unfamiliar with, because there isn't much I have not been taught, researched, or tried. So they are always very encouraged and can focus on the actual progress of their programs.

Most of my clients feel an immediate change in their energy and body when they incorporate some of these supplements along with the nutrition plan. It is truly magical. I know this might sound weird and you may even think, how can this be, but I honestly felt better during my cancer protocol than before I even had cancer. And I have many clients who feel the same way when they change their nutrition and add in supplements to their daily regime.

Take Donna. She had Type 2 diabetes, and was taking metformin and insulin. She came to me because her physician said she needed to be on these two meds in order to control her diabetes. She didn't want to be on medicine. She was frustrated because she was working out, but couldn't lose weight and didn't feel well. She had heard about all the great success my clients were having with diabetes, so she decided to work with me.

When she first came to see me, she said she felt defeated and exhausted, lacked ambition, had terrible cravings and headaches, and was feeling bloated most of the time. She was also starting to feel depressed. I told her that I thought that by making dietary changes, lifestyle changes, taking a few key supplements, and changing up her exercise program, she would probably be able to be completely off her medications in a few weeks, and that she would start to feel better pretty quickly.

Most of my clients just need a little help and a little coaching to turn their lives around, change how they feel, and reverse disease. Donna was no different. After only two months working with me and slowly titrating off of her meds, she was able to stop taking them completely. Her Type 2 diabetes was gone. She was no longer bloated, her body was responding, and she was losing weight. Her cravings were gone, her headaches rare, and her emotional health was restored. She no longer felt depressed; she felt alive again. Just think if she would have listened to her doctor and continued on the metformin and insulin drugs! First of all, if she would have continued on her insulin drugs, she probably would have become insulin resistant and in many cases the type 2 diabetic loses pancreatic function almost completely over time and begins to resemble type 1, which means she would be insulin and medication dependent forever. She would have continued to feel frustrated, unhappy and unhealthy. Instead, in just two months, she reversed her diabetes.

For me? Nine months. It took nine months for me to heal my lymphoma. That's incredible. You can do this, too. You can reverse your disease and take action on your health. Now, after months of being cancer-free, I feel absolutely fantastic. I finally gave my body what it was strongly asking me for. I am living my REFUSED Solution. I can't wait to get you on it, too.

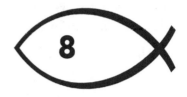

E — ELIMINATING STRESS

"Do not be anxious about anything, but in every situation, by prayer and petition, with thanksgiving, present your requests to God. And the peace of God, which transcends all understanding, will guard your hearts and your minds in Christ Jesus."

– Philippians 4:6-7

Around the seventh month of doing my holistic protocol and being rigorous with my nutrition, supplements, and daily detox routine, I started getting yeast infections. Like, a lot. I had never had them before. I didn't understand why I was suddenly getting them, and it started to freak me out. So, of course I tried to learn why. I instantly looked up yeast infections and cancer. Oh, boy…. This was the start of a downward spiral. I convinced myself that these infections had something to do with my cancer, and even though I treated them with an anti-fungal, they'd come right back.

Shortly after that, I started not feeling well. I was having pressure and pain in my neck at the incision point where I'd had surgery. I was also experiencing pressure in my right arm, and having pain in my chest and lungs. I was continuing to get yeast infections. I was terrified that maybe my protocol wasn't working and my cancer was growing back. I had been monitoring my progress this entire time with Dr. Conners. Doc would test me and say I was fine, the pee test was coming back with lower numbers. Oh, and by the way, when I say the pee test was coming back with lower numbers, I'm referring to a specific urine test that detects the number of abnormally dividing cells in your body, which is how I tested the entire time and one way I knew I was improving. This test is a great non-invasive, cheap, and effective way to measure progress.

So everything seemed to be going great, as hoped. But, deep down, when I started to not feel well, I questioned myself and I questioned my protocol. I would think to myself, "What if it's not working? Why do I have pain in my chest? Why is my neck feeling weird? Is my lymphoma spreading to my chest?" I was having the worst negative thoughts.

My decision to use natural methods was always, always my first option, and I was very confident in trying it. I was 100% convinced I was doing the right thing. There was too much evidence, proof, stories, and data to support reversing my cancer. So what changed? Month seven, WORRY kicked in. Once I let the worry take over my thoughts, I was on a downward spiral, mentally. I questioned everything. Why was I starting to not feel well? Why did I have pain in my chest and lungs? Had it spread to my chest? Why was I now getting yeast infections? Was I growing new cancer?

I would check every day to see if I had any new lumps. I was working myself up to the point that there were days when I couldn't even relax and my chest pains would get worse. I didn't share this with anyone except my husband. He kept telling me, "Teri, you are totally fine. You are healed, I truly believe it." Although these words were comforting to hear, I wanted to believe that in my heart. But for the first time in seven months, I was doubting.

In month nine, I went to see my doc, and I brought Mark with me. I told Dr. Conners about my symptoms and that I was concerned. I asked him what he thought might be going on. He checked me and said I was fine, but noted that I appeared anxious and stressed out. I told him I was scared because I haven't been feeling well for a couple months, dealing with these symptoms were really scaring me, and I needed hardcore proof that this was working.

Dr. Conners said, "Teri, it is working, but in order for you to have peace of mind, you should go have a PET scan."

But I didn't want to do a PET scan. I didn't want to put radioactive sugar in my body, nor did I want to be exposed to more radioactive scans. My husband and Dr. Conners both said that they really felt I needed peace of mind. Honestly, I was scared. Part of me wanted to know, but part of me didn't. What if? What if?

After that appointment, and after my husband and Dr. Conners encouraged me to get a PET scan, I decided to face my fear and do it. I really didn't want to expose myself to a PET scan, but I also wanted to have proof. Proof what I was doing was working. I wanted to prove to my oncologist that she was wrong and my way would work. But, deep down, I was scared. Really, really scared!

On December 29th, three days before the end of the year, I went in for the PET scan. I had to do it before the end of the year so my insurance would pay for it. The day before, I had to eliminate all sugar, drink lots of water, and pretty much only eat protein.

PET scans, by the way, are horrible. It is a nuclear imaging scan that shows disease in your body. They first inject radioactive sugar and dye into your body, and make you drink barium. Then you lie on a table, and the combined matching of the CT and PET scan images are taken. If tumors or disease are present, the radioactive sugar circulates throughout the body and will accumulate in the tumor because cancer loves sugar. If you have cancer, you will light up like a Christmas tree.

When I got to the clinic, the tech explained what she would be doing and what to expect. She said I wouldn't feel anything and that it was an easy process and blah, blah, blah. They injected the radioactive sugar and dye. It felt hot, I could feel it entering in my bloodstream. I drank the barium. Yuck. Gagged it down, and it made me nauseous. About an hour later, I started to get a pounding headache. Oh, no….

After the scan, I got in the car and was terribly sick. My head was pounding. I got home and started throwing up right away. This lasted for a day and a half. On Friday, the 30th, I was lying in bed, still sick and with a migraine, when Mark barged into my room to ask me if I heard from the oncologist about the results. I said that I hadn't, that I'd been in bed all day with a pounding headache and throwing up, I had no idea whether or not they'd called. Mark was not happy with that answer. All I could think of was how sick I felt and how scared I was to find out what was going on. I felt horrible.

The next thing I remember was Mark coming up to the bedroom with his phone in his hand and telling me to wake up … wake up…. He proceeded to play a message he'd recorded of him and the oncology nurse talking.

> Nurse: "From the results of the PET scan, it shows that Teri has no disease in her body."
>
> Mark: "Can you say that one more time?"
>
> Nurse: "Yes, the PET Scan shows that Teri has absolutely no disease in her body."
>
> Mark: "Oh, that is great news! I love you and you don't even know it yet!"
>
> Nurse: (Giggling) "Glad I could give you such great news to kick off your new year."

AND THAT, MY FRIENDS, WAS THE NEWS OF A LIFETIME!!!!

Words cannot explain the instant joy, relief, and gratitude that flooded my soul. It was a feeling like I'd never had before in my entire lifetime. I was absolutely amazed, in awe, and grateful. I cried and cried, I got down on my knees beside my bed and thanked God. God healed me, He healed me. I praised Him and thanked Him and all my tears were of joy. It was a feeling that I remember vividly to this day. I get teary-eyed every time I recall that moment. It was a huge load lifted off of me. In fact, the next day, the *very* next day, I no longer had chest pain. Gone! Ha. Funny how that works, huh? How many of you are so chronically stressed out that your body is giving you physical signs? Time to start paying attention.

The worry that I allowed to overtake me for two months had manifested into physical symptoms. Let me say that again. I had myself so worked up into a stressful, worrisome tizzy that my chest pains, pressure, and symptoms were all related to the worry, and it all started with some silly yeast infections I was getting due to teaching cycle class and not changing my clothes immediately afterwards, *not* from cancer. I convinced myself I was not healing. Ai yi yi. What a huge lesson for me.

What Is Stress?

Let me give you an education on stress. Stress is a killer. Stress will ruin you and make you sick. There is a strong link between stress and cancer. Many studies have connected stress with suppressed immune function and disease. Disease feeds off stress, which comes in mental/emotional form, physical/biomechanical form, and chemical/biochemical form.

Mental/Emotional: This is any form of anger, worry, anxiety, bitterness, unforgiveness, frustration, insecurity, nervousness, depression, shame, jealousy, and any other negative emotion.

Physical/Biomechanical: A stress of some sort of trauma to the body, such as when we have surgery, break a leg, are in chronic pain, or are out of alignment.

Chemical/Biochemical: A physiological stress, such as toxicity, nutritional deficiency, hormone imbalance, parasites, viruses, and funguses.

All of these forms of stressors cause reactions in the body that keep our bodies inflamed. Stress also has two types: acute and chronic. Acute stress is a short burst of stress, like if you are running from danger, or escaping a fire, something really stressful in a short period of time. Chronic stress is day in, day out emotional, physical, or chemical stress that keeps your stress hormones elevated for a long period time.

So let me give you a little physiology lesson. Cortisol and adrenaline are the two hormones that surge from our adrenal glands when we are in a stressful situation. The stress can be physical or emotional or chemical. Your body doesn't know the difference between a stressful day at work, you being chased by a robber at gunpoint, or you having a parasite. It's just going to try and figure out how to fix it.

Cortisol is released by converting glycogen to glucose in the liver, and then it goes to your bloodstream to give you energy. Adrenaline is the hormone that will give you power or strength to fight off an attacker, or to run faster, or get out of danger. So these two are working together to give you energy and power for what your body perceives to be an emergency. But like I said before, if you have a bad emotional thought, you are still going to release these hormones just like you would if you are being chased by a bear. They are doing their job, but they are supposed to be released in those times of a real emergency. The other thing is that when cortisol and adrenaline are released, they switch off other body functions that are not needed in a short-term, life-threatening situation. When these stress hormones are continuously being released, it is very damaging to the immune system.

When you have all these kinds of stressors going on in your life, it is very damaging and has many negative implications. If your body is in constant state of urgency, that state is perceived hormonally as a threat, so your body automatically does things to protect itself. When trauma goes unhealed or unresolved, the body system is in a continual state of urgency. There have been findings that the sympathetic nervous system (SNS) can cause cancer metastasis when it is chronically activated. The SNS is the part of the body that is responsible for releasing adrenaline and noradrenaline which "turn on" and cause genetic alteration if we never give our SNS a break. If our SNS is always turned on (meaning we are uptight, stressed out) all the time, then many things start to happen. Here are some ways stress (the hormones released) can lead to cancer. Remember, the human body doesn't differentiate between a major stress or a minor stress. Regardless of the situation causing the stress, the body is reacting by:

✓ Shutting down our immune response

✓ Causing inflammation

✓ Reducing the function of our natural killer cells

✓ Inhibiting apoptosis

✓ Hindering DNA repair

✓ Causing new cancer stem cells to form

✓ Increasing the chance of angiogenesis

✓ Promoting obesity due to elevated cortisol and insulin resistance

✓ Shutting down digestion processes so you are unable to absorb nutrition

I bet that as you are reading this, you can identify with the stress you have in your life. I have talked to a lot of cancer patients, and every single one of them shared with me that they have had major stress in their lives. Many I spoke with were, like me, undergoing a traumatic experience or significant life stress during the period leading up to the day they were diagnosed. If you are under stress and do not work to get hold of it, you will not be able to heal your cancer. If you don't manage the stress hormones in your body, your own immune system can't fight for you. You *must* recognize the areas in your life that are stressful and make every attempt to work on a strategy for creating less stress. Getting a cancer diagnosis is very upsetting. I understand. This is something I had to really work on. I know for me, once I understood that the chances of me healing my body naturally were way healthier and more likely to work than doing chemo and radiation, I felt far less stressed. I instantly could start to relax about my treatment. I honestly cannot imagine the horrific stress a person who undergoes chemo must have.

Once I had that managed, it was a matter of controlling all the other areas of my life that I knew were causing me stress. I had to tackle them immediately, and come up with a game plan. My understanding of the relationship between stress and cancer was very clear. I know my years of chronic stress are what contributed to my lymphoma. I am 100% convinced of that, and so was my holistic doc. You see, I am a type A, driven person. I am always pushing myself. I am a perfectionist and people pleaser.

Here is another really interesting fact about emotional stress and cancer. Dr. Ryke Greerd Hamer confirmed anatomical brain changes in patients with symptoms of cancer. His findings and principles solidly base the nature of disease on universal biological principles and on the interaction between the three levels that make up the organism: the psyche, the brain, and the organ. His study indicates that certain root causes of stress are related to certain types of cancer and physical symptoms. For example:

- ✓ Your opinion is disrespected = lung/head and neck cancers

- ✓ Love betrayal/relationships/marriage and divorce = breast cancer/ovarian/prostate cancers

- ✓ Anger = liver cancer

- ✓ Taken advantage of or feeling disrespected by family, friends, or colleagues = stomach, colon, renal, and bladder cancers

- ✓ Intellectual disrespect = brain cancer

- ✓ Perceived as carrying the weight of the world = musculo-skeletal cancer

- ✓ Perceived as being ugly = skin cancer

- ✓ Perceived lack of public recognition = pancreatic cancer

The years of stress I have put my body through have not helped my health. I am totally convinced that my stressful lifestyle is what suppressed my immune system over the years and caused my cancer to develop. Being an entrepreneur brings about many joys and blessings, but also stress and hardship. Being a one-woman show for my business caused me to work long hours, deal with a multitude of difficult people, work through challenging financial times, not get enough rest, not take enough time off, say "yes" to too many things, and aim for perfection. The first time I got the message my body was stressed, was when I was diagnosed with adrenal fatigue. My second message? Cancer. Got the message, loud and clear.

Cancer, for me, was a huge wakeup call. I had to control my stress. I had to learn how to manage it better. I had to give my body the emotional relief (unite with God), physical relief (more sleep) and nutritional relief (get rid of all toxic loads) it needed to reverse the cancer in my body. And where I needed to do the most tweaking was my stress.

This was and is my true challenge. Food and nutrition — easy. Environmental toxins — easy. Daily detoxing — easy. Taking my supplements — easy. Uniting and spending daily time with God — easy, but still growing and learning. Eliminating stress? A huge challenge.

You are probably reading this and thinking all of these are hard for you. They should be … you didn't know. But now that you are reading this book and have more knowledge than ever before, you can take the steps needed in order to make whatever necessary changes to get you on the right track. Remember, I have been there. I am always here to help you along the way.

How to Manage Stress

Here is how I manage my stress. First and foremost:

Spend daily time with God. He gives me strength, guidance, and understanding. This is really my only source of true peace. If I'm not connected to Him daily, I have stress. If you have unresolved emotional wounds or have any toxic relationships that are consuming you, you have to get those resolved. If you have lingering bitterness, fear, or negativity in your life and you don't address it, everything you are doing in your healing protocol can be outweighed by your stress. I truly could not do this without God's help. But whatever your belief system is, if you don't resolve these, you will continue to keep your body in a state of stress that will inhibit you from healing your cancer.

You can try meditation and visualization, which is very helpful for many. I am a huge fan of Joyce Meyer. She is my spiritual mentor. Honestly, if it weren't for her messages, videos, and devotional lessons, I think I would have struggled a lot more. God has used her to help me. I connect with her on a spiritual level, and that also helped me cope with my own life. I would love to meet her someday. If anyone can hook me up, please do. Ha! My point is, you really need to find someone to whom you can relate to on a spiritual level and be committed to digging deep into your spiritual journey. This will help with your mindset, and in order to have healing success, you have to have a positive mindset.

Exercise. There is a direct link between exercise and regulating our stress hormones. Daily walking, aerobics, weight lifting, rebounding, or whatever physical activity gets you moving is important for a healthy body and stress reduction.

Laugh it off. Laughter boosts your immune system. I surrounded myself with laughter and positive conversations, and I watched funny movies and TV shows. I didn't engage in toxic conversations or friendships. I had to fill my mind with fun and laughter. Turn off the news, and quit watching shows that are making you feel upset. If social media is making you stressed and it is causing negative or unhappy feelings, stay away or cut way back — and for Pete's sake, delete or unfriend anyone who is not bringing value or joy to your life. Surround yourself with positivity.

Sleep. I changed my schedule so I could sleep in. I rarely wake up to an alarm clock anymore. I listen to my body and sleep as much as I can. I will say this: Before I was on my anti-cancer protocol, I was tired all of the time and wanted to daily take naps. Now, because I sleep better and longer and put good nutrition in my body, I don't feel the need to nap. I have great energy all day long.

Lastly, I prayed this prayer and others like it daily, to keep me from feeling the overwhelm.

> *My Stress Prayer: Lord, I recognize that I have allowed my stress to take control of me. I need your help. I cannot continue to live stressed out and anxious. I want to change, I really do. Need your help. Give me insight, help me make changes that will alleviate my stress in life. Help me to laugh things off, learn to relax, not over-react, and enjoy life to its fullest. Thank You. Amen.*

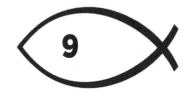

D — DETOX

"Most people have no idea how good their body is designed to feel."

– Kevin Trudeau

L et me tell you about Pam. Pam was a smoker. She was a client who really wanted to break the smoking habit, lose weight, and become healthier. She was not feeling good. She had low energy, she was coughing a lot, had trouble sleeping, and a difficult time working out due to her smoking addiction. She was also very constipated; she was only pooping about once a week. Yikes, that is just not right. It is a very bad situation if you are not eliminating daily, which I will talk to you more about in a little bit.

Pam got started on some daily changes that would allow her body to naturally detox and clean out her colon. This consisted of changing her nutrition, implementing an exercise program, and adding some cleansing supplements. She really needed to try to start detoxing her body from all of those toxic cigarettes. She also decided she was going to quit smoking cold turkey. I put her on a one-week colon cleanse that consisted of specific foods, some herbal supplements, fiber, herbal teas, sauna, and exercise.

After four days, she was in a panic and said that her poop was solid black. She was concerned, but I knew that this was the tar and nicotine being excreted. Her body was so caked with nicotine that we ended up having to do back-to-back cleanses. Eventually, her poop returned back to its normal color, and she was finally pooping every day. Her energy was better, and, the best news of all, her cravings for cigarettes were greatly reduced, making it a lot easier for her to quit cold turkey. Her body was starting to eliminate the toxins. When you have toxins in your system that you do not detoxify, it can create a lot of damage to your cells, liver, and organs. You will notice a host of symptoms and, eventually it can turn into disease. Pam was amazed at the change in how she felt and was thrilled she was finally able to quit smoking.

This is how powerful detoxing, supplements, and holistic approaches are in creating homeostasis in the body. Our bodies want to be healthy, we just have to be able to provide them with the right conditions in order to repair the damage that we have done.

Detoxification is really misunderstood. Most people think that you can just use a 10-or 20-day detox kit that is packed with supplements and water only, and then you'll be totally detoxified. This is so far from the truth. Most of these detox kits don't work, are a waste of money, and do not teach you the most important thing about detoxing, which is this: *stop using and eating things that are toxic*. You must learn what you are doing that is making you toxic.

You must decrease your toxic load. Basically, stop toxifying your body by what you are doing, eating, wearing, and breathing. We should be detoxing every single day and reducing the toxic load that causes our bodies to become stressed, inflamed, and sick.

Let me explain the ways our body detoxes, and then we'll talk about how to do this.

Our liver is our main detoxification organ. The liver and kidneys detoxify our blood. These two organs work together to keep our blood clean. They filter out all the metabolic waste and toxins that enter our bodies through what we eat, breathe, or put on our skin. They work every day to get rid of the toxins as well as clean our blood and lymphatic fluid. If your toxic load gets too high, your liver and kidney get clogged up, and then your detoxing pathway is not going to be working, which is why you get sick.

Your lungs are another detoxing organ. Every time you inhale, you are cleaning your blood. Every time you exhale, you are excreting toxins that have been converted to carbon dioxide. Deep breathing alkalizes, promotes detoxification, and oxygenates your entire body.

Your skin is another way you detox. Your skin is your largest organ, so when you sweat, you are eliminating numerous toxins. It is super important that you sweat, your body needs this in order to maintain your health and get rid of harmful toxins.

Elimination. The last way your body detoxes is when you go to the bathroom. I know, I know, most of the time people don't want to talk about this, but if your pee is dark yellow and you are not pooping daily, you are not detoxifying. The more you poop, the more you are detoxifying.

Now let's talk about some of the methods that are most effective in detoxing your body.

First and foremost, you have to make sure you are not putting toxins *in* your body. This is what you are exposed to in your environment (Chapter 4) and what you are eating (Chapter 5). You have to make your first priority to work on the E and F in the REFUSED Solution if you plan to set yourself up for successful daily detoxing. If you are eating foods that are packed full of GMOs, or you are eating foods that are sprayed with fertilizers and pesticides, or are smoking and breathing in toxins, you can't expect your body to keep up with the heavy toxic load. Our bodies really do try and keep up, but when they get saturated with toxins and our liver and kidneys can't keep up with the demand, they get clogged and wear out, causing disease. And we are exposed to an enormous amount of these chemicals every single day. Hopefully you have learned a few things and will decide to clean up your food and environment so you can allow your body to function properly.

Here are the top detox methods that I used to cure my cancer.

Exercise

There are so many health benefits to exercise, that I could write a book just on the amazing benefits to your mental and physical health. When my clients ask if they should be exercising every day, I ask them, "Do you want to be in a good mood every day?"

Obviously, if you have cancer, the ability to exercise may be challenging, but if you can, you really need to make this a part of your anti-cancer protocol. Exercise helps you to detox. You have three times more lymphatic fluid in your body than blood.

Blood pumps through your body via a pump, and is continuously moving. Your lymph fluid is thick and does not move if you don't move. The lymphatic fluid is like butter. When you warm up, it gets thinner, when you cool down, it thickens up again. Your lymphatic system's primary job is to remove toxins, metabolic waste, and dead cellular debris through the body where it can be eliminated via urine, sweat, liver, mucus, and poop.

Exercise is the most effective way to improve this function. Any exercise that you can do that allows you to heat up that lymphatic fluid, sweat, and move, is going to be very beneficial in detoxifying. One of the absolute best forms of exercise for your lymphatic system is rebounding. Rebounding creates a G-force that stresses every cell in your body in a positive way. It promotes the circulation of the lymphatic fluid, which again is thick and not as fluid as your blood. Rebounding is also low-impact, so it is really a great way to get exercise. I made it a priority to either exercise with aerobics, spin, weights, or rebounding every single day when fighting my cancer. Exercise also increases the oxygen supply to all your tissues and cells and stimulates the circulation of your blood.

Sweating

Sweating is an effective way to cleanse the body and eliminate waste via the skin. Exercise has this benefit also. But what I think is absolutely the most relaxing way to sweat is sitting in an infrared sauna. I love, love, love infrared saunas. Let me tell you, not only are they super relaxing, but the health benefits go far beyond just sweating. Based on research studies, infrared sessions reduce risk of cardiovascular disease, lower blood pressure, increase blood flow, improve skin texture, reduce wrinkles, help with eczema and psoriasis, increase the body's resistance to infection, stop virus replication, and reduce chronic pain. Sitting in an infrared sauna is extremely relaxing and has a calming effect on the nervous system. I cannot speak highly enough about infrared sauna treatments. Unlike a traditional sauna, the infrared rays act directly on the body and not on the air. This allows the rays to resonate through the dermis up to two inches deep, which allows up to six times the amount of toxins being extirpated as compared to traditional saunas. When you sweat like this, you are excreting heavy metals, toxins, and unwanted acids and strengthening the immune system as well as enriching the tissues with oxygen. So, you want to make it a habit to sweat, if not via a sauna, for sure with exercise.

Daily Elimination

There is no polite way of saying this, but you have to be pooping every single day. If you are not pooping, you are storing and recirculating toxins in your body. It is very common for cancer patients to be constipated. Actually, it's not just cancer patients, it's everyone. You should be pooping a minimum of once per day. Ideally, one to three times per day. It is very common that a new client will tell me that they haven't gone to the bathroom in days. There are many reasons why someone may be constipated. Could be what they're eating, hormone imbalances, lack of exercise, dehydration, medications, stress, or internal medical issues, but the main reason my clients are constipated is due to their nutritional choices. If you eliminate GMOs, eat organic food, increase your daily consumption of fruits and/vegetables, increase your fiber, and eliminate meat, you will set yourself up for better digestion, absorption, and elimination. It is painful to be constipated. It is also extremely toxic and can lead to colon cancer and other types of cancer. It is important to make sure you are pooping every single day. I am an expert in constipation. Yeah, it's true. Mainly because the majority of women who come to me wanting to feel better, are chronically constipated. Over the years, I have had to learn the many different reasons why they are constipated and have been able to figure them out, therefore, making me the constipation guru... I guess... ha.

Deep Breathing/Getting Oxygen

Cancer cells hate oxygen. Hmm, say what? Again, exercise is a source of getting oxygen to your cells. But what is the reason why deep breathing is important? It helps clean your blood when you breathe in. When you breathe out, you are excreting toxins. Deep breathing alkalizes, oxygenates your entire body, and promotes detoxification. So right now, as you are reading this book. I want you to take a deep breath in. Hold ... and blow out. See, didn't that feel nice? You should make this a habit and do it a few times a day. I would do this while sitting in my infrared sauna. You are deep breathing while exercising, so take the time to try and make this a daily habit.

I also wanted to understand why oxygen was so key in killing cancer. So when I was researching this, I learned that high oxygenated environments are toxic to cancer cells. I learned about Hyperbaric Oxygen Therapy (HBOT). The Hyperbaric Oxygen Chamber is a tube that you lie in that is filled with pressurized oxygen. Hyperbaric oxygen therapy (HBOT) is the medical use of oxygen in a pressurized environment used to saturate the blood plasma (blood cells), which leads to a broad variety of positive physiological, biochemical, and cellular effects. One is that it slows down the growth of cancer cells and triggers cell death. When oxygen is administered at high pressure rates, up to 20 times more oxygen can be absorbed by the bloodstream. Hyperbaric oxygen slows cancer growth, boosts the supply of circulating stem cells, promotes the growth of new capillaries and blood vessels, stimulates oxygenation, supports wound healing, and increases the survival rates in patients with metastatic cancer by 77%.

I wanted in on this. It made sense to me, and I wanted to do whatever I could to provide an environment where my cancer would not grow and I wanted to kill cancer cells off. Otto Warburg was a world-renowned cell biologist and cancer researcher. He discovered that cancer cells exhibit an abnormal metabolism and cannot thrive during cellular respiration. Cancer cells are low in oxygen primarily because they have changed from taking in and utilizing oxygen for respiration to a more primitive form of respiration that utilizes sugar instead of oxygen. It is the cancer process itself that causes most of the lack of oxygen, not the lack of oxygen that causes the cancer process. If you Google Otto Warburg, you will see all of his scientific research on this topic. I sat in a Hyperbaric Oxygen Chamber for an hour about four or five times per week.

Fasting

Fasting is a really effective way to get your body equipped for immediate detoxing. Although I would always recommend incorporating nutritional changes first if you have cancer, there are definitely periods of time when a person should consider fasting. Fasting allows and helps your body to heal and repair. Fasting helps to supercharge your immune system. When you give it a break from digesting food, it allows the energy that would normally have been used for digestion to be able to upregulate the immune system in order to use its energy to switch from digestion and focus on the operation of repair and healing, encouraging white blood cells to eradicate dormant infections such as cancer growth. Fasting also increases the breakdown of damaged, old, and toxic cells. Fasting also improves insulin sensitivity. Cancer cells have a lot of insulin receptors, so when you fast, it deprives the cancers cells of its fuel and maintains proper blood sugar levels.

There are different ways to fast. You can do water fasts or juice fasts, and vary the length from one day to five days. You can do intermittent fasting daily, or for a period of time. It all depends on your situation, and it's best to check with your doctor, of course, before you do this, but the benefits of fasting are very effective for many reasons, especially targeting cancer growth.

Coffee Enemas

I know this sounds absolutely horrible, but it is one way to remove toxins that are stuck to the colon, improve gut motility, increase energy levels, improve constipation, and reduce toxicity in the entire body by promoting liver cleansing. What happens when you do a coffee enema is that the coffee instantly goes to the liver to secrete more bile, which stimulates detoxification. Coffee enemas also promote the production of a powerful antioxidant produced by the liver called glutathione. It is a powerful antioxidant that protects cellular damage and stimulates the removal of toxic waste out of the cells. Anyone with cancer will benefit from doing these.

Supplements

There is a reason why I put supplements as the very last detox method. Although I believe in supplements, a person has to change their food and fix their environment first. I know I sound like a broken record, but if those two things aren't addressed first, then the use of supplements is just going to be a big waste of your money. The supplements will work best if you create the environment where they can actually be absorbed, utilized, and work. DNA testing will help you learn how your body is able to detox and what pathways are not working to their fullest potential. In that case, there will be specific supplements that you will need for your own DNA. I mentioned a couple detox foods/supplements in Chapter 7, but here are some very effective ones that could be incorporated immediately.

✓ Chlorella — is a heavy metals detoxifier.

✓ Spirulina — inflammatory and targets cancer stem cells and eliminates tumors

✓ Cilantro — rids body of heavy metals like arsenic, aluminum, lead, and mercury

✓ Broccoli sprouts — very powerful liver detoxing food

✓ Milk thistle — helps prevent and repair liver damage

✓ Probiotics — I could do an entire chapter on the importance of pre-and probiotics, but they are imperative for digestion and immune function. Also, they facilitate the proper elimination of waste.

✓ Burdock root — clears toxins from the blood and detoxifies the liver. Also helps with lymphatic drainage and detoxification.

Rife Machine

Used for detoxification and killing cancer cells, the radio frequency of this machine can target bad cells in your body that are responsible for other health complaints. The Rife machine proved that specific radio frequencies can destroy invasive microbes and unwanted growth cells without adversely affecting the body's tissue or cell structure, and without harming the good bacteria in our system. This is because every molecule actually resonates at a specific frequency, and by isolating the frequencies of toxins and bad bacteria, only they are affected by the Rife machine's radio waves. This is why an opera singer can break a wine glass without hurting anybody or anything else around it. Dr. Rife isolated 52 frequencies that could be used to destroy certain unwanted cells.

Royal Raymond Rife was a brilliant scientist who created the very first microscope that was able to actually see a live virus. Rife was able to see live bacteria and live viruses in a person's blood sample. He identified the human cancer virus first in the 1920s.

So the concept is that with cancer, by using a Rife machine, you can match the frequency of the type of cancer that you have, and kill that cell by hitting the frequency of that organism. By using a light frequency generator, Rife discovered he could manipulate and kill the pathogens, viruses, and bacteria. It also alkalizes the tissue by raising the ph. So the Rife machine is a great tool to bring homeostasis back to the body on a cellular level.

In Dr. Conners' book, he explains that once the pharmaceutical companies took over the medical industry, all of the cancer doctors who were not using pharmaceutical drugs were run out of the country. When Rife was shut down and all of his equipment destroyed, he gave up. The AMA did its job. They were out to destroy anyone or anything that was in competition with them. The FDA today does not recognize this technology as an accepted treatment method (of course not), so it falls under the category of alternative healthcare.

But the fact is, when Royal Rife was conducting his cancer studies, he had a 100% cure rate of all the cancer patients he tested that used the Rife machine. You won't ever hear about this, but if you go and read up on it, you will see this is the case. Now you understand why the Rife machine is not promoted in the cancer clinics. Its success rate is too high in curing cancer. According to Dr. Conners, everyone who has cancer should be using a Rife machine as part of their cancer protocol.

As you can see, daily detoxing can become a permanent lifestyle once you understand what you need to do. Even though I cannot specifically tell you how these will work if you are doing chemo and radiation, because that was not the route I chose, I can say that with all of my studying, research, and working with Dr. Conners, everything in the REFUSED Solution will be beneficial and useful even if you are undergoing chemo and/or radiation. In fact, it will be important to incorporate these to your protocol to ensure a better outcome and hopefully fewer side effects.

All of these methods are going to be important to do as you fight your cancer. You must exercise, sweat, breathe, and poop daily. These are also going be actions that you want to make a habit. I can speak for myself and tell you that all the cancer survivors I have spoken with were doing almost all of the above detox methods. Once they started to clean up their nutrition and environment and made it a daily ritual to exercise, sweat, poop, and breathe, they noticed positive changes immediately.

Fighting cancer is about knowing what your body is designed to do, and then giving it what it needs in order to function properly. If you have cancer, your immune system is damaged and its ability to kill the cancer is suppressed. I wondered how in the world someone like me, as a health and fitness guru, and years of nutritional background could get cancer. Well, I think I figured it out. My stress was high, my nutrition was not ideal, and my immune system was suppressed. I am way more educated now about all of the things that contributed to me getting cancer. Knowing this and being able to change it is so powerful and empowering. It is so comforting to know that I am doing everything I can to keep my body fighting this disease. If I can keep my stress under control, I should live a long, healthy, and cancer-free life.

I can only imagine what you are feeling right now. You are probably encouraged, but yet feeling really overwhelmed and maybe need to set the book down and go get a hot tea to give your brain a rest. Here is what I want you to try to let sink in. Something is better than nothing, and starting is better than procrastinating. Healing cancer is very similar to healing obesity. It takes time and there is no quick fix. You will need to try numerous things, not all at once, of course, but you will have to try many methods. You also have to be consistent. Don't expect to try something for a week and then go off for two weeks, and then try again for another week. You can't lose 100 pounds in one week, but you can lose 100 pounds in one year. During that process, you start small, by lifting light weights and exercising to your body's own ability. You also have to make changes with your nutrition. You know you won't lose that 100 pounds if you don't change what you are doing.

Losing weight is hard. Curing cancer is hard. But both are doable. And in both cases, there is no quick fix. You have to start somewhere: be consistent, continue to try different things, find support, monitor your progress, and stay optimistic. Detoxing is critical in both losing weight and fighting cancer.

I cannot wait to visit with you, because together we will identify what detox methods you should start with and why. You will be as thrilled as I was when you start to feel better and incorporate some of these detoxification protocols.

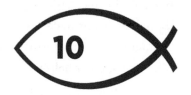

GET YOUR POWER BACK

I can do all things through Christ who strengthens me."

– Philippians 4:13

will never forget the time I was having a conversation with someone who I really looked up to. He was a medical doctor, and I was looking forward to sharing with him what I had been doing for my holistic treatments for the past 12 weeks. I shared with him that my cancer marker numbers were lowering, which was a very good thing. When I was telling him, he was acting aloof and very disinterested. I took this as his way of showing me that he was not in agreement with what I was doing. I remember him telling me that there was no scientific proof that what I was doing was working and I could tell that he doubted that my numbers were actually going down. I mean, blatantly not believing me. Seriously? He thought I would lie about something like this or make this up? It was more important for him to interject his uninformed opinion versus encouraging me or offering me other helpful feedback.

Instead, he proceeded to tell me that he had a patient with cancer who was trying holistic. He said he didn't think she was going to make it, because he thought she should be doing chemotherapy, and not dabbling in holistic nonsense. I asked him what his patient was doing and how she was testing herself. He said she was doing some supplements, but also at the same time on a diet that her oncologist put her on. He said she was not doing well and was probably going to die.

First of all, what part of holistic was he talking about if she was following the nutritional advice of an oncologist? We already know that they know nothing about nutrition. How naive! I have seen the diet plans that oncologists give to their patients. They consist of high-sugar protein drinks, lots of white processed foods, and GMOs. I'm quite certain his patient was dabbling in the holistic world, but was probably not working with anyone other than her oncologist and was not getting any help. If she was "all in" with holistic, she wouldn't be listening to what her oncologist told her to eat, by any means. I was so annoyed with him, I just walked away and decided to never talk with him again about my situation. When he learned that I was cancer-free, he didn't even congratulate me or say anything.

Here were some of the other comments I received, unsolicited, when some people learned I was going a different direction other than chemo.

COMMENT: "Teri, you really should do chemo and radiation. You don't want to take a chance with treatments out there that are not proven to work. I know of many people who have had chemo and survived."

MY THOUGHT: Yah, but, I don't just want to survive, I want to LIVE. I want to cure my cancer. I have seen how people who "survived" cancer really lived life. They were suffering, in pain, and now have many awful long lasting side effects. I do not want that.

COMMENT: "You don't want to mess around with cancer, Teri, chemo is the treatment that you should do."

MY THOUGHT: How do you know it is what I should do? Have you researched both sides? Do you even know how successful the holistic treatments are?

COMMENT: "Teri, you'll get through it. You're the strongest woman I know. You'll fight this and kick its butt."

MY THOUGHT: It's so easy for you to say. I know I am strong, you are right. I am strong and smart enough to know that I can fight this a healthier way, but you are not the one having to fight it.

COMMENT: "You have so many friends and clients that will support you and won't care that you lose your hair."

MY THOUGHT: I don't want to be bald. I don't want to look sick, oh Lord, I can't do this.

COMMENT: "Eventually, you will learn to laugh while doing your chemo treatments. You can have a chemo party and wear your favorite hat and serve refreshments and turn them into a party."

MY THOUGHT: Really? Are you being serious right now? Chemo parties? What part of chemo is worth celebrating? I certainly do not want to celebrate chemo. That is not my kind of party. What the??

COMMENT: "You know my uncle died of lymphoma, he suffered for years and it kept coming back."

MY THOUGHT: Sheeesh, thanks so much for sharing that uplifting news with me. That is really encouraging and great for me to hear right now.

COMMENT: "From what I understand, chemo and radiation are pretty effective in treating lymphoma."

MY THOUGHT: Ok, and from what I understand, and what makes total common sense to me is, if chemo and radiation are "supposedly" successful in treating lymphoma by putting poison in your body, then why wouldn't putting healthy treatments in your body also be successful?

COMMENT: "I wouldn't do that if I were you". (Meaning holistic treatment)

MY THOUGHT: Well, you are not me.

COMMENT: "You know, they make wigs look so realistic these days."

MY THOUGHT: Then you go buy one for yourself.

COMMENT: "Don't worry, you have tons of people that will help you and step in for you when you're sick."

MY THOUGHT: I don't have time to be sick, I don't want to be sick in bed all day and not be able to teach my classes and have fun with my friends. This is not the quality of life I want to live.

What the Wha? Yes, I swear, these were some of the things that people said to me. Talk about stressful! When you get diagnosed with cancer, I swear, some people turn into complete insensitive jerks. I am sure many don't intentionally mean to make you feel bad, but when you are told the worst news of your entire life, the last thing you want is people's negative opinions. Either way. You want empathy, support, and positivity. Talk about stressful. You will have a lot of naysayers, pessimists and strongly opinionated people coming at you when they find out you have cancer. If you decide to do chemo and radiation, you will have people saying you shouldn't without even knowing why you shouldn't. If you decide not to do chemo and radiation, you will have people who say you are really stupid for not getting medical treatment and trusting your oncologist. You can't win. It is so important that you follow the steps laid out in this book before you make a decision either way.

Some of the Common Obstacles to Your Success

Even on your best quest to figure out how you are going to heal your cancer, you will have many obstacles. There will be times you will want to quit. I did. I remember one day being down because I had gotten another medical bill in the mail that pertained to the first surgery that I had where they removed the wrong gland. I was thinking I have no energy to fight it. At the same time, I was all out of my holistic supplements that I needed, and I was due for a checkup appointment with my holistic doctor, none of which was covered by medical insurance. I had to come up with another $900 to continue the protocol, treatments, and appointments. I remember at that moment wanting to quit. The financial burden was a lot to bear most days.

Financially, it was tough, very tough for us to go the holistic route. But I wouldn't do it any other way, NO WAY! We found a way to make it work. It was and still is a financial thorn, but the alternative options (medical coverage for chemo/radiation and meds) are not the better options for your physical or mental health, that's for sure.

Instead of wanting to quit during the difficult moments, I am encouraging you to take these times and use them to learn, grow, and become stronger. I can honestly say, and I know you might not believe me, that I am thankful for my cancer. My cancer changed me. It has given me a whole new perspective on life, it's given me better friendships, way more inner peace, improved health, and most importantly, it grew my relationship with God. Thanks to cancer, I feel like a new person. A disease that could have killed me actually gave me new life, though not without some challenges along the way. The challenges made me stronger, gave me new perspective, and taught me patience and faith.

Thinking Your Oncologist Is God

You will be pressured, you will feel torn, you will feel conflicted. Cancer is a multi-billion dollar industry. Your oncologist will push you pretty hard to do their treatment. Mainly, because, quite honestly, this is the only treatment they are taught. I don't think all oncologists are evil, but I do know that they are not being told the truth nor are they being shown the holistic cures that are out there. This is not their fault (entirely), but they will push you hard to use chemo and radiation. I can think of two reasons why you would be more likely to turn to allopathic cancer treatments. One, they are scaring you to death and telling you that you might die if you don't use their conventional treatments. Also, your oncologist says that chemo drugs and radiation are the only method of treatment that is going to work to put you in remission (remember, it's never called a cure). Two, you haven't researched holistic for yourself or met with a holistic doctor to get their treatment advice.

Medical Insurance

This is a huge, huge obstacle. It's such a medical scam; it makes me sick. If I had chosen chemo and radiation, my insurance would have covered it entirely (with a $10,000 copay, of course), but to go to a naturopath doctor to get holistic treatments and supplements meant insurance covered nothin'. Zero, zilch, $0. Holistic treatments range anywhere from $10,000 up to $100,000 or more based on what kind of cancer protocol plan you have in place. So you can totally understand the dilemma. It is something that is a huge problem for many cancer patients.

Negative Story Tellers

You will have people that will be so open to sharing with you a story about their friends/acquaintances who had cancer and give you the horrific details of their experience. I am sure you have heard one or more of these comments from your circle of friends. If it hasn't happened yet, it's coming. Your family and friends are worried about you. They care about you, but they are uneducated. They don't know what you know.

Hopefully after reading this book you are feeling more empowered and are closer to taking the steps you need to heal your cancer. But, I am telling you, you are going to get criticized. You are going to be pressured to do things the ways that others are wanting you to do them. The pressure will be so strong that you will start to doubt yourself and your decisions. This is inevitable. But getting your power back, doing your research so you are strong in your decision about your healing protocol, will get you through these times.

Family/Friends Not Supportive

Andrew has colon cancer. He decided not to do chemo and radiation. He is very committed to learning what he can to take a holistic path of healing. He is getting pressure from his mom. His mom is telling Andrew that his son needs to see his dad around in five years. This makes Andrew feel conflicted. He loves his son. He loves his mom, too, but his mom is putting a lot of pressure on Andrew to change his mind. She is scared, for him, of course, but the constant pressure from his mom is making him second guess himself. He also works in construction. He used to be a bodybuilder, so he looks fit and in shape. He is athletic, attractive, and has a strong work ethic. He is afraid he is going to lose his construction job if he is sick all of the time. If he loses his job, how will he support himself and his son? He doesn't want his friends to see him sick. He cries when he tells me that he pictures himself going from a muscular build to a skinny, unhealthy, and bald dude. He doesn't want to be co-dependent on others. He wants to continue being active. He is scared his cancer will spread. He is afraid to die. He understands he needs to surround himself with other cancer success stories and be a part of the REFUSED Solution. He needs the support, structure, and reminders of what he knows to be the best decision for him. He realizes that if he unplugs from the solution, he will not have enough support to continue to be accountable to the steps.

Your immediate family will be the people who will push against you the hardest, if you decide to not go with the traditional cancer treatments. Again, this is only because they don't know what they don't know. This is why you must educate yourself first and then educate them next.

Fear Your Treatment Isn't Working

Fear is a daily occurrence when you have cancer. And it doesn't help that others want to check in on you every day and subliminally make you question what you are doing. Fear is an emotion with cancer that you have to learn how to manage. Fear sneaks in and tries to make you doubt yourself. Every day, you are wondering if it's working. You will find that, even going through the REFUSED Solution, you will have days of fear, doubt, and uncertainty. You will have weird symptoms of your body healing and you will think it's more cancer. You will have some pretty icky detoxing side effects that are really a good sign of your body healing, but you will freak yourself out and think it's something else. Every ache, pain, or twinge will be alarming. You will be overly sensitive to everything.

Doing This on Your Own Sucks

In each and every conversation you have with your friends and relatives during your protocol, you will wish you could tell them you are healed. Doubt becomes very evident when you don't have anyone to support your decision and stand beside you. Having others in the REFUSED Solution Program will give you the support you need. Also, you will have me to help keep you accountable to your end goal, which is to heal your cancer. Also, not having anyone to talk to about your progress or symptoms is unsettling. There will be days when you just want to talk with someone who really understands what you are going through. Unless you have or have had cancer, no one can truly share your experiences. Your faith, spirit, morale, and decisions will be tested. Having others who can help you, keep you accountable, and guide you on the right path needs to be a huge priority. You might experience frustration, impatience, and doubt the entire process.

Here is the good news: I've gone through all of these challenges and come out on the other side with a great healing story to share and teach you. It's the best feeling. I had a clean PET scan after nine months of using the REFUSED Solution. If anyone understands all of the objections and negative emotions you are and will be going through, it's me. I get you! I understand! I want to help you through the process. You do not have to go through this alone and confused. I will help you get through this. Going through this with others who understand will be a whole lot better than going through it alone. It will be worth having the support and ability to talk with others who are in the same boat as you are.

CONCLUSION

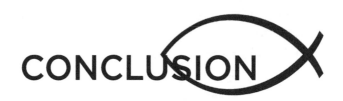

"They that wait upon the Lord shall renew their strength; they shall mount up with wings as eagles, they shall run and not be weary, and they shall walk and not be faint."

– Isaiah 40:31

I believe in you. I care about you. I have faith in you and this process. You will make the best decision for you, I know you will. You know why I know this? Because I have prayed for you. Every reader of my book has been prayed over. This is why I know that whatever you decide, will be the best decision for you.

My strong desire and message in this book is this. You have time. Time to s-l-o-w down. S-L-O-W the entire process down and do your due diligence to learn, research, and understand everything you can before you decide on a plan of action. When I say S-L-O-W down, I mean right out of the gate. The day you get diagnosed, start researching. Meet with your oncologist with the intention to learn as much as you can about your situation. Try not to let them scare you into getting started with their treatment right away. Be prepared to ask them a lot of questions, interview them, to see if you are comfortable with their handling of your health. Hopefully after reading this book, you will be more equipped to ask the hard questions and stay calm and more confident during the appointment. Slowing down and taking some time to digest everything after reading this book, will give you power! You will feel so much more in charge once you take the power and become your own health advocate. My hope is that this book will provide you with a solution you can try first, before you decide to do chemo and/or radiation.

But on the other hand, I also need to say this. I do understand my entire book has been about how I REFUSED chemo and radiation, and my position is a very strong one. But I also need you to hear me on this. If you decide that chemo and radiation is what you must do, even after reading this book, then that is your decision. You have to stand behind it and just make sure it was a well-informed decision made by *you* and not your oncologist, family members, friends, or others. Here is the good news. If you do decide to do chemo and/or radiation, then the REFUSED Solution will be a *must* for you. You will be doing things to support the immune system, and each of the steps in this book are going to help you during your chemo treatments. It will be imperative that you give your body the support it needs while undergoing those treatments.

My hero, mentor, and friend, Dr. Conners (who wrote the foreword for this book) will agree that even if you decide to use chemo and radiation, your chance of success and healing are going to increase with the use of the REFUSED Solution. Dr. Conners has treated many patients who have used or are using chemo while working with him, and he has seen better results with the patients who abide by the methods described in this book. Of course, my hope for you is that you choose to use holistic alternative protocols to heal your cancer. But as much as I desire that for you, you have to be the one who, after reading this book, is convinced that holistic is the direction you want to go. If that's you, I cannot wait to help, guide, and coach you through what I know is going to be the most challenging time of your life.

Of course, my dream for you is that your cancer will change you for the better, like it did me. That you will be healed and have the peace of mind of knowing that when you heal your cancer from the inside out, you don't have to worry about it coming back.

Having this confidence is, in itself, worth more than anything. When I was healing my cancer, the only thing I wanted was 1) to be healed, 2) to have peace that it would not come back, 3) that I would learn from it, be changed by it (grow spiritually and mentally), and 4) that I would be an amazing example to others; by being able to help, serve, and support others during this difficult time.

My hope is to be able to offer insight, encouragement, love, support, and to help present options to you so you can become your own health advocate. My dream came true. This! I pray your dream will come true, too. This is the reason I wrote this book. For you, my dear friend. I love you, and I am here to serve you in whatever way that I can.

FURTHER READING

Cancer Free: Guide to Non-toxic Healing — Bill Henderson

Beating Cancer with Nutrition — Patrick Quillen

Cancer Revolution — Leigh Erin Connealy, MD

Stop Fighting Cancer and Start Treating the Cause — Dr. Kevin Conners

Life, Cancer and God — Paula Black and Capt. Dale Black

The Truth About Cancer — Ty Bollinger

Radical Remission — Kelly A Turner

The China Study — T. Colin Campbell, Thomas M. Campbell

Outsmart Your Cancer — Tanya Harter Pierce

Overload: How to Unplug, Unwind, and Unleash Yourself from the Pressure of Stress — Joyce Meyer

RESOURCES

AARC Publications. "Dietary Flaxseed Alters Tumor Biological Markers in Postmenopausal Breast Cancer." http://clincancerres.aacrjournals.org/content/11/10/3828.short

BFit Challenge. "No to GMO's." https://blog.bfitchallenge.com/?s=gmo

BFit Challenge. "Mystery Solved: No more bloating!" https://blog.bfitchallenge.com/2016/10/22/mystery-solved-no-more-bloating/

Budwig Center. http://www.budwigcenter.com/

Cancer Treatment Center of America. "Non-Hodgkin Lymphoma Stages." http://www.cancercenter.com/non-hodgkin-lymphoma/stages/

Centers for Disease Control and Prevention. "Vaccine Excipient and Media Summary." https://www.cdc.gov/vaccines/pubs/pinkbook/downloads/appendices/b/excipient-table-2.pdf

Centers for Disease Control and Prevention. "Possible Side Effects from Vaccines." https://www.cdc.gov/vaccines/vac-gen/side-effects.htm

Collective Evolution. "Chlorine in Water Could Be Linked to Human Cancers." http://www.collective-evolution.com/2013/08/15/chlorine-is-toxic-what-you-need-to-know-about-chlorine-your-health/

Connealy, Leigh Erin. The *Cancer Revolution: A Groundbreaking Program to Reverse and Prevent Cancer.* De Capo Press, January 2017

Connett, Paul, et al., "Revisiting the Fluoride-Osteosarcoma connection in the context of Elise Bassin's findings: Pt II", submitted to the NRC review panel on the Toxicology of Fluoride in Water, April 8 2005.

Conner's Clinic. "Genetic SNP Testing." http://www.connersclinic.com/genetic-snp-testing/

Consumer Reports. "Talking Turkey: Our new tests show reasons for concern." http://www.consumerreports.org/cro/magazine/2013/06/consumer-reports-investigation-talking-turkey/index.htm

Crosswalk. "Faith Produces Resilience: Daily Hope with Rick Warren, Dec 29, 2015." http://www.crosswalk.com/devotionals/daily-hope-with-rick-warren/faith-produces-resilience-daily-hope-with-rick-warren-dec-29-2015.html

Dr. Axe. "10 Flax Seed Benefits and Nutrition Facts." https://draxe.com/10-flax-seed-benefits-nutrition-facts/

IARC Monographs. Chemical Agents and Related Occupations. http://monographs.iarc.fr/ENG/Monographs/vol100F/mono100F.pdf

Ion-Cleanser. "The Rife Machine for Detoxification." http://www.ion-cleanser.org/the-rife-machine-for-detoxification.html

Livestrong. "What Are the Benefits of Amla Powder?" http://www.livestrong.com/article/280952-what-are-the-benefits-of-amla-powder/

National Cancer Institute. https://www.cancer.gov/research/areas/causes

National Geographic. "Marine Pollution." http://ocean.nationalgeographic.com/ocean/explore/pristine-seas/critical-issues-marine-pollution/

NCBI. "Targeting treatment of cancer with artemisinin and artemisinin-tagged iron-carrying compounds." https://www.ncbi.nlm.nih.gov/pubmed/16185154

NCBI. "Risk of human ovarian cancer is related to dietary intake of selected nutrients, phytochemicals and food groups." https://www.ncbi.nlm.nih.gov/pubmed/12771342? dopt=Abstract

New Medicine. "Review of The Germanic/German New Medicine of the Discoveries of Dr. Ryke Geerd Hamer." http://www.newmedicine.ca/overview.php

Science Daily. "Science News: How inflammation can lead to cancer." https://www.sciencedaily.com/releases/2011/04/110419091159.htm

TBYIL (The Best Years in Life). "Oxygen and Cancer -What Warburg Actually Discovered." http://www.tbyil.com/Warburg_Oxygen_Cancer_Tony_Isaacs.htm

The Truth about Cancer. "Medical Mafia: Buyer Beware or Buyer Be Dead." https://thetruthaboutcancer.com/medical-mafia-buyer-beware-buyer-dead/

The Truth about Cancer. "Quest for the Cures", 2014 Video. https://thetruthaboutcancer.com/charlene-bollinger-talks-about-the-quest-for-the-cures/

The Truth about Cancer. "Fluoride — Drinking Ourselves to Death?" https://thetruthaboutcancer.com/fluoride-drinking-ourselves-to-death/

The Truth about Cancer. "The Façade of Breast Cancer Awareness, Susan G. Komen and the Pink Ribbon." https://thetruthaboutcancer.com/susan-g-komen-pink-ribbon-facade/

The Truth about Cancer. "The Healing Benefits of Hyperbaric Oxygen Therapy." https://thetruthaboutcancer.com/hyperbaric-oxygen-therapy/

Vaccine Injury Info. "Vaccines and the Immune System." http://www.vaccineinjury.info/vaccinations-in-general/vaccines-and-immune-system.html

VaxTruth. "Vaccine Facts." http://vaxtruth.org/vaccine-facts/

VaxTruth. "Vaccine Ingredients: A Comprehensive Guide." http://vax truth.org/2011/08/vaccine-ingredients/

Vaxxed: From Cover Up To Catastrophe (video) http://vaxxedthemovie. com/

Whale. "2-phenoxyethanol (2-PE)." http://www.whale.to/a/ phenoxyethanol.html

Wired. "News Break: FDA estimates US livestock get 29 million pounds of antibiotics per year." https://www.wired.com/2010/12/news-break-fda-estimate-us-livestock-get-29-million-pounds-of-antibiotics-per-year/

ACKNOWLEDGMENTS

Thank you to:

My husband. I love you. You are my rock. Thank you for your unending support and patience, help, and prayer. I understand being on the other end of this was not easy for you. I thank God for you every single day.

Dr. Conners. Thank you for your wisdom, discernment, expert advice, and spiritual insight. You truly are the most intelligent human being I know. I thank God for bringing you to me and using you to help me through the most difficult time. There was a reason for us to meet.

My parents. You kept me encouraged. Your support was without judgment. You were at appointments and surgeries, and your daily prayers and calls meant more to me than you know. Thanks for your financial help, spiritual help, emotional help, and unending love.

Darla. You gave me strength when I was at my weakest. Your words touched my soul. They lifted my spirit on some of my darkest days. I felt your prayers, your concern. For you, I will always be grateful.

Women of BFaith. You were the first to know of my cancer diagnosis. Thanks for letting me share my personal journey with you all. Your prayers, notes, gifts, flowers, and words of encouragement helped me feel loved on days when I needed to feel loved. Our strong connection to each other through prayer and support means the world to me.

My clients, past, present, and future. I wouldn't be where I am today without you. I have learned so much from all of you. I will continue to be a student. This book is for you. I am so honored that you chose me as your coach, and my commitment to you is to always serve you with integrity, love, and wisdom.

Cancer. You no longer scare me. You came to me at the perfect time. I thank you for changing my life forever. Because of you, I have learned so many valuable lessons. Because of you, I will now serve everyone I meet even more deeply from a servant's heart. You broke me only to make me stronger. For that I am thankful.

My Heavenly Father. Dear Lord. I love you. I praise you. I honor you. Without you, my life is nothing. You healed me. You taught me and continue to teach me life's most important lessons. I am so thankful for my renewed relationship with you. Thank you for speaking to me on days when I wanted to give up. Thank you for allowing me to see the bigger picture. My desire for anyone reading this book is to be blessed and touched by you. I wrote this book because I was led to. I wrote this book to first and foremost share my story. My story of how you changed me for the better. Lord, please touch the hearts of everyone reading this book. My desire is that you use *me* and this book for your glory, always and forever.

To the Morgan James Publishing team: Special thanks to David Hancock, CEO & Founder for believing in me and my message. To my Author Relations Manager, Gayle West, thanks for making the process seamless and easy. Many more thanks to everyone else, but especially Jim Howard, Bethany Marshall, and Nickcole Watkins.

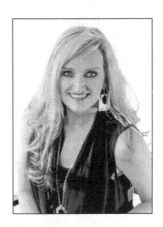

ABOUT THE AUTHOR

Teri Dale is a functional diagnostic nutritionist, cancer coach, weight loss expert, life coach, and author who has committed her life to helping others transform their health. When she was diagnosed with Hodgkin's Lymphoma, her world turned upside-down, but her experience will inspire you and teach you that cancer does not have to feel like a death sentence. Teri was able to beat her cancer in nine months and created a solution in facing this horrible disease. Teri is passionate about helping others who are suffering in any way. She strongly believes that any challenge in your life can change you, if you are willing to face it and learn from it. She has been in the health and fitness industry for over 20 years and owns a transformation studio and coaching business helping women transform their lives. Teri lives in Minnesota with her husband of 13 years and her adorable Pomeranian, Gus. Connect with Teri by email at teri@teridale.com or visit her website at www.teridale.com, www.irefusedchemo.com and www.facebook/irefusedchemo.

THANK YOU

Congratulations on taking the time to learn and under-stand what it is going to take to heal your body from disease. I hope you have done some of the action steps that I suggested throughout the book, and that you already feel more encouraged, empowered, and less alone.

I am excited to help you. To help you on your way to get-ting your power back, becoming healthier, confident, and more fit. Let me invite you to enjoy my free 7-day course on the REFUSED Solution. Now that you have completed reading this book, go to www.irefusedchemo.com and opt in for your FREE 7-day course. I look forward to meeting with you someday and helping you on the inside.

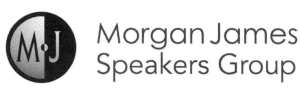

Morgan James
Speakers Group

↗ www.TheMorganJamesSpeakersGroup.com

We connect Morgan James published
authors with live and online events
and audiences who will benefit
from their expertise.

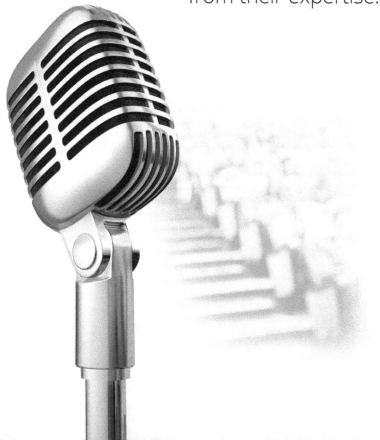

Morgan James makes all of our titles available through the Library for All Charity Organization.

www.LibraryForAll.org

Printed in the USA
CPSIA information can be obtained
at www.ICGtesting.com
JSHW022343140824
68134JS00019B/1663